MALTREATMENT AND THE SCHOOL-AGE CHILD: DEVELOPMENTAL OUTCOMES AND SYSTEM ISSUES

Phyllis T. Howing, MSW
John S. Wodarski, PhD
P. David Kurtz, PhD
James Martin Gaudin, Jr., PhD

SOME ADVANCE REVIEWS

"The authors engage in a wide-ranging critique of existing practices and policies toward children and families in the social service, education, mental health, and juvenile justice systems and make recommendations for sweeping changes. They argue persuasively that . . . social programs must be established to help repair the damage already done; damage that is eloquently chronicled in this volume. Social workers, teachers, and court and medical personnel who work with children must be aware of this information and alert to the special needs of abused and neglected children."

Kristine E. Nelson, DSW, MSW
Director of Research, The National Resource Center on Family-Based Services; Associate Professor, School of Social Work, The University of Iowa

"A major advance in understanding how maltreated children develop during the school-age years. The authors provide illuminating case vignettes in many chapters, bringing to life the numbers. The closing chapters describe some of the limitations of the current mix of service systems and offer useful suggestions for improving existing efforts to prevent and respond to child maltreatment. Should be in any library dealing with child maltreatment."

Robert Schilling, PhD
Associate Professor, School of Social Work,
Columbia University

"An important book because of its pioneering efforts to assess the long-term effect of physical abuse and neglect on school-age children and to differentiate between the sequelae of the two types of maltreatment. Many practitioners find research studies murky and incomprehensible. The easy-to-read style, case examples, and careful craftmanship of this volume make it an exception and one that should be well-received."

Joan W. DiLeonardi, PhD
Executive Vice President, Childrens Home & Aid Society of Illinois

---

NOTES FOR PROFESSIONAL LIBRARIANS AND LIBRARY USERS

This is an original book title published by The Haworth Press, Inc. Unless otherwise noted in specific chapters with attribution, materials in this book have not been previously published elsewhere in any format or language.

CONSERVATION AND PRESERVATION NOTES

The paper used in this publication meets the minimum requirements of American National Standard for Information Sciences–Permanence of Paper for Printed Material, ANSI Z39.48-1984.

Maltreatment and the School-Age Child

Developmental Outcomes and System Issues

HAWORTH Health and Social Policy

Marvin D. Feit, PhD
Senior Editor

New, Recent, and Forthcoming Titles:

Maltreatment and the School-Age Child: Developmental Outcomes and System Issues by Phyllis T. Howing, John S. Wodarski, P. David Kurtz, James Martin Gaudin, Jr.

Maltreatment and the School-Age Child

Developmental Outcomes and System Issues

Phyllis T. Howing, MSW
John S. Wodarski, PhD
P. David Kurtz, PhD
James Martin Gaudin, Jr., PhD

The Haworth Press
New York • London • (Norwood) Australia

The Haworth Press, Inc., 10 Alice Street, Binghamton, NY 13904-1580

Library of Congress Cataloging-in-Publication Data

Maltreatment and the school-age child : developmental outcomes and system issues / Phyllis T. Howing . . . [et al.].
p. cm.
Includes bibliographical references and index.
ISBN 1-56024-291-4 (acid free paper).
1. Abused children–United States–Psychology. 2. Abused children–Services for–United States. 3. Child development–United States. I. Howing, Phyllis T.
HV741.M338 1993
362.7′68′0973–dc20 92-1205
CIP

In memory of Dr. Jeanne Odell

ABOUT THE AUTHORS

Phyllis T. Howing, MSW, Project Coordinator at The University of Georgia School of Social Work, coordinated the research project discussed in this book. The co-author of numerous journal articles on child abuse and neglect, she has served as a board member of the Athens, Georgia Council on Child Abuse and facilitated a Parents Anonymous group.

John S. Wodarski, PhD, is Professor of Social Work for The University of Akron, Ohio. The author of two hundred referenced publications and nineteen texts, he has presented hundreds of papers at conferences and professional societies and organizations. Dr. Wodarski serves on review panels for The National Institute of Child Abuse and Neglect and The National Institutes of Health.

P. David Kurtz, PhD, Professor of Social Work and Education at The University of Georgia, is a licensed clinical social worker. His expertise includes working with troubled children and adolescents and their families. Dr. Kurtz has directed many research projects and recently acted as Principal Investigator of a juvenile justice study. He is a member of the National Association of Social Workers and the Georgia Council on School Social Work.

James Martin Gaudin, Jr., PhD, is Assistant Professor and Director of the Research Center for the School of Social Work at The University of Georgia. He is the author of numerous publications on the subjects of child neglect, social networks, and incarcerated mothers. Dr. Gaudin is currently Principal Investigator for a study of family structure and function in neglectful families for the National Center on Child Abuse and Neglect.

CONTENTS

List of Figures

List of Tables

List of Case Profiles

Appendix

Foreword

Few books so vividly present the results of top-rate social science. The authors set out to learn the shared and distinct fates of older children who have been neglected and physically abused. The authors' combined clinical and research sensitivities are evident in the study's design and implementation. The choice of questions about family functioning, social status and support, services, and child functioning demonstrates a commitment to building information useful to practice and policy. Selection of the best available research strategies and measures shows respect for the challenges of child abuse research.

Child abuse researchers and practitioners are sitting on top of a rapidly moving enterprise in which there are far more unknowns than knowns. We have come to accept the fact that child abuse is related to stress and social isolation; more controversial are notions that child abuse is related to socioeconomic status and race (the counterpoint to this argument is that child abuse *reports* are related to socioeconomic status and race). Still less understood and debated is the way that social class, stress, and race are related to child abuse and its outcome. The authors address these difficult relationships in an intriguing chapter that considers family background characteristics, type and chronicity of maltreatment, and foster care placement.

Research on outcomes of child maltreatment must also consider the quality and appropriateness of intervening services. The authors examine services provided in the home and foster care services. The findings on foster care are particularly provocative and illuminating but not positive. My own research and practice convinces me that, although foster care provides vastly underestimated good to thousands of children every year, it has often been a "whipping boy." Yet, this book's unusually close look at the experiences of youth in foster care convinces me of the urgent need for better foster care.

The book does not allow us to continue deluding ourselves that effective children's services are only needed for infants and toddlers. In the 1980s, the age of children receiving child abuse and child welfare services dropped swiftly. With escalating numbers of child abuse reports, the children's services system moved to investigating and serving only the most immediately vulnerable young children and victims of sexual molest; if an older child could run away or fight back to protect herself, she was too often on her own. This volume clearly shows how great and lasting the vulnerability can be for older maltreated children. At the same time, the work shows the resilience of many youth (if they are given some support). If we fail to fashion programs to redress the enduring harms of neglect and abuse for these children and provide opportunities for renewal, we will awake each day with our shame and walk each step toting a heavy social and economic burden. The nation should apply this strong tonic of realism to the development of additional services for promoting the educational and social well-being of abused children–regardless of age.

The authors have applied much effort and skill to distilling a clear product from an enormous array of information. Authors generally understand that the more sources of information used, the richer the understanding can be. These authors obtained information from parents, teachers, social workers, and the children themselves; after they collected it they went back and collected more to assess change; they found a comparison group of children who could help highlight the unique contribution of the maltreatment to development. More challenging, and rarely executed as well as in this volume, is the integration of all those sources of information so readers can clearly visualize the lives of children and families, the current social response, and the alternatives. The authors have done this with a blend of strong writing, carefully chosen and placed statistical information, and case materials.

The volume uses case material to illustrate the complex interplay of background, abuse, and service factors that determine children's current performance. The cases are not just attention grabbers; they are treated substantively. Each one includes a discussion of family stressors, indications of socioemotional and academic functioning from the assessment battery, a service profile, and a depiction of the current status of the child. Most illustrative is the discussion of how the child's individual story can explain current outcomes as well as the fit between the child's experience and that of the general study sample. These discussions both bring poignancy to the research findings and provide an exemplar of the intricacies of applying study findings to practice with abused children.

The distillation of information is not done at the cost of overgeneralization. The authors have taken great pains to distinguish the academic and socioemotional outcomes for the physically abused, neglected, and sexually abused children. Their findings call our basic assumptions and practices into question. The book is about child maltreatment, but not only maltreatment. More general child development and social policy implications become clearer as each page is understood. The findings regarding the effects of social class, family stress, and educational responses on children are applicable to a wider group of children.

The authors bring significant research and practice expertise in child welfare service, mental health, education, and juvenile justice to their endeavor. So, when they call for better integration between these systems, they command the understanding and the mastery of details needed to go from rhetoric to action. The interventions the authors recommend are specific to each strand of children's services but also address the cross-cutting issue of integrating these services.

This book brings us the latest in child abuse research and yet, in a curious way, is a throwback. In this increasingly pressured era, most research is generated in the form of journal articles that can be submitted along with quarterly research reports. If you want the full impact of an important research project, you must put it together from 12-page pieces or, if you are lucky, the author(s) may more thoroughly discuss sets of findings from their study in a book chapter. This is hardly the way to make a significant statement. Few authors now take the time to develop their work into book-length treatments that can serve as lasting resources for methodology and content. This volume follows in the tradition of other book-length studies on child welfare that have significantly shaped our response.

This volume leaves no doubt that we must not forget the hundreds of thousands of older maltreated children in the child welfare service system. This important book clarifies ways that we can assist these children by fundamentally changing the response to them. From their findings, the authors draw clear implications of severe educational detriments among their neglected sample and of serious socioemotional harms for their physically abused sample. By tracing life histories, the authors understand the ways that allied services have left these children unprotected and unprepared. The book does not demand that the reader work hard at deciphering research findings–those are clear as a bell. It *does* emphatically insist that the reader work to find ways to provide improved services for maltreated children and all children. The volume goes well beyond cursing the darkness to cast considerable light on ways to proceed toward a new era of child abuse science and service.

Richard P. Barth
Berkeley, California

Preface

What happens to children whose parents beat them or fail to provide the essentials for survival? Research confirms that failure-to-thrive babies wither in the absence of mother bonding; that abused toddlers hit their playmates; and that maltreated preschoolers and kindergartners show an alarming array of social, emotional, and cognitive problems. But few researchers have examined the consequences of parental abuse or neglect on the school-age child.

This book addresses that gap by presenting the findings and implications of a major research project on 8- to 16-year-old maltreated children. Our results show that these children suffer severe damage that current child-serving systems are ill-equipped to repair. Yet, without appropriate interventions, many of these children seem destined for failure as students, workers, parents, and contributing members of our communities.

It is no small problem: Nationwide, nearly 1.5 million children are identified as physically abused or neglected every year, and the true incidence is undoubtedly much higher.[1] The problem is not going away, and it will never go away if disregard for the plight of children in our society continues. We hope this book will provide new awareness and insight for all readers, new ideas for those who work with older maltreated children, and fresh ammunition for those who speak out on children's issues.

The first two chapters discuss prior research and how this study was designed and carried out. The concepts in these chapters (and the entire book) are presented in lay person's terms and, we hope, catch the sense of purpose, immediacy, and absorption that attended the project as it took shape. Chapters Three through Six present specific findings on the academic, socioemotional, and functional development of the children and characteristics of their families and backgrounds, along with implications for treatment. The final two chapters explore deep-rooted system inadequacies and propose remedies that can help prepare older maltreated children for successful adulthood and parenthood.

The authors wish to gratefully acknowledge the outstanding assistance of personnel from the Departments of Family and Children Services and the school systems that participated in our project. Without their generous contribution of time and effort, neither the project nor this book would have been possible.

We also appreciate the excellent feedback and support provided by Richard Barth, Byron Egeland, Joan DiLeonardi, Kristine Nelson, Robert Schilling, Jim Whittaker, and our colleagues and graduate assistants at The University of Georgia School of Social Work. Special thanks go to Ken Gauger, Phyllis Westbrook, Kathy Burgraff, Shary Karlin, and Karen Gill for their technical assistance. Finally, we give thanks for funding provided by the National Center on Child Abuse and Neglect (grant No. 90CA136/01); The University of Georgia Office of the Vice President for Research; The University of Georgia Research Foundation, Inc.; and The Hazen Foundation. Portions of this book were previously published in *Social Work*.[2]

NOTES

1. National Center on Child Abuse and Neglect, *Study Findings. Study of National Incidence and Prevalence of Child Abuse and Neglect: 1988* (Washington, DC: U.S. Government Printing Office, 1988).
2. J. S. Wodarski, P. D. Kurtz, J. M. Gaudin, Jr., and P. T. Howing, "Maltreatment and the School-Age Child: Major Academic, Socioemotional, and Adaptive Outcomes," *Social Work* 35 (1990): 506-13.

Chapter One

The Gap in Child Maltreatment Research

Over the past two decades we have learned a great deal about the consequences of abuse and neglect for the developing child. A substantial body of research provides abundant evidence of cognitive, social, and emotional problems in young maltreated children. So far, however, researchers have focused their efforts almost entirely on infants, toddlers, and preschool children. Much less is known about the consequences of abuse or neglect on the older child, although older children are at greater risk of maltreatment.[1]

While children of school age (elementary to high school) may be less likely than younger children to die or require hospitalization as a result of neglect or injuries inflicted by parents, we cannot doubt these children are damaged by maltreatment. Evidence that older maltreated children are strikingly overrepresented in populations of runaways, delinquents, truants, teenage mothers, and substance abusers suggests that the consequences of abuse and neglect are indeed serious for these children.[2] However, no study has ever presented clear evidence of a causal link.

An understanding of the specific effects of abuse and neglect on the older child is of critical importance when establishing sound policies and practices for dealing with these children. Professionals, who are required by law to report suspected maltreatment, and Child Protective Services (CPS) workers, who are charged with substantiating these reports, are hindered by our inadequate knowledge base. These gatekeepers may misclassify children if they are not aware of the developmental deviations that appear in the older maltreated child. Interventions are more likely to be effective when they address the specific social, emotional, academic, or functional problems found in these children. Further, in order to more effectively apportion the limited funds available for addressing social problems, policymakers at all levels must have an understanding of the specific consequences and costs to society that result from the maltreatment of older children.

To address this gap in our knowledge, the National Center on Child Abuse and Neglect commissioned the University of Georgia School of Social Work to conduct a study of school-age children who were physically abused or neglected. Over the course of the project, 69 maltreated children aged 8 to 16 were compared with 70 nonmaltreated peers on a wide range of developmental and family factors. A vast amount of information was gathered about these children and their families from parents, foster parents, teachers, caseworkers, school records, and the children themselves. Some 2,500 questionnaires were filled out, and over 500 interviews were conducted over a two-year period. The information has now been examined in depth, and profiles of the older abused or neglected child have emerged.

This book presents the project's findings. It is written from the researcher's standpoint, with the researcher's respect for data, methodology, and tests of significance. However, since our findings are of general interest and have broad social implications, we have eliminated research jargon wherever possible and provided simplified explanations of research procedures, terms, and concepts likely to be unfamiliar to lay persons.

Not surprisingly, we found marked delays in the development of abused and neglected children and striking differences between maltreating and nonmaltreating families, but some of our most provocative findings showed unexpected strengths in these children and their families. In later chapters, we will explore specific findings, describe specific cases (omitting identifying information), and examine current policies and practices that affect school-age maltreated children. The first two chapters focus on background factors and research concepts that are essential to an understanding of our findings. To design an effective study, we first had to consider a range of theoretical constructs, research findings, and child welfare system practices.

WHAT IS CHILD ABUSE?

The phenomenon of child abuse has only recently come to widespread public awareness. Two decades ago the topic was rarely mentioned. Now, cases of children who have suffered or even died from maltreatment flood the media and it has become clear that children who survive maltreatment are damaged in many ways. The tremendous increase in reports of child abuse and neglect reflects the public's growing concern over the problem. The fact that more than half of these reports are labeled "unfounded" after investigation[3] indicates that there is some confusion about what constitutes officially recognized maltreatment. Most often, unfounded cases are not considered serious enough to warrant intervention.

Under current working definitions of maltreatment, physical abuse means more than a spanking or whipping, and neglect means more than living in poverty or being a latchkey child. The abused and neglected children we studied were victims of serious maltreatment. These children had sustained burns, welts, bruises, and other injuries inflicted by parents; or they had suffered from lack of essential food, shelter, medical care, or protection by parents.

This study focused on physically abused or neglected children, not children whose primary classification was emotional maltreatment or sexual abuse. Emotional maltreatment, which may involve such distorted parent behaviors as habitual verbal assault, rejection, tying a child to a bed, or confining a child to a closet, is extremely difficult to detect and substantiate. Thus, official intervention in these cases occurs far less often than in physical abuse and neglect cases.

Cases of sexual abuse have increased rapidly over the past decade, but still account for fewer than 10% of identified maltreatment cases.[4] Widespread awareness of the problem is so recent that standards for sexual abuse research may not yet be rigorous enough to establish the effects of this form of abuse. Studies have not consistently controlled for such factors as the nature of the abusive incident (e.g., fondling vs. rape), the seriousness of the child's injuries, the relationship of the child to the perpetrator, and the separate effects of the intervention process itself (intervention in physical abuse and neglect cases is generally much less disruptive to the child). Thus, confusing and contradictory findings have been reported which suggest, probably erroneously, that sexually abused children sustain only moderate emotional (and no academic) damage.

Although we did not focus on sexual abuse, some of the children studied had either experienced this form of maltreatment in the past or in conjunction with recent physical abuse or neglect (in no case was sexual abuse considered the primary problem). Thus, we were able to make a rudimentary assessment of the effects of sexual abuse on these children. Not surprisingly, we found almost no differences based on sexual abuse, but we must emphasize that this may reflect the methodological problems referred to above rather than a true lack of effect.

MALTREATMENT AND CHILD DEVELOPMENT

We hypothesized that the children who had been abused or neglected would be developmentally delayed compared with their nonmaltreated peers, and that this delay would be evident in various measures of school performance, social and emotional development, and functional behavior.

School Performance

The upper limits of our intellectual capacity may be genetically predetermined, but there is no guarantee that we will fulfill our intellectual potential. Environmental factors may conspire to rob us of our birthright. Cognitive development is a dynamic process, and our later academic performance in school is dependent upon abilities developed step by step through earlier experiences. Numerous studies confirm that fundamental learning processes are critically affected by our early environment. A child who is nurtured and encouraged is able to master each new learning task at the appropriate age and move on to the next. Children who are raised in environments that are low in intellectual stimulation and parental warmth, or high in parental control and harsh discipline, are likely to be slow in developing speech, perception, memory, and thinking abilities.[5] Thus, it comes as no surprise that young children who have been abused or neglected show quite significant delays in intellectual functioning, typically scoring 10 to 20 IQ points lower than their nonmaltreated peers.[6]

We might expect the abuse or neglect that occurs during the school years to have quite a different effect on intellectual development than that which occurs during the critical preschool years. A child who has already mastered the fundamental learning tasks of the early years certainly has a head start in meeting later cognitive tasks. However, the rate of mental growth for the individual child is characterized by plasticity; IQs may rise or fall significantly throughout childhood and adolescence depending on environmental factors.[7] For the school-age child, maltreatment would be expected to interrupt concrete and abstract reasoning abilities that normally develop during these years, and these lags inevitably would affect school success.

Of course, maltreatment of an older child may have been preceded by years of less-than-optimal parenting, if not overt abuse or neglect. Thus, cognitive delays may already be established by the time the child reaches school-age. Furthermore, poor school performance can reflect more than cognitive impairment. Intellectually capable students may fall behind academically because of social or emotional problems that interfere with classroom performance.

Socioemotional Development

The extensive literature on children's normal social and emotional development repeatedly emphasizes that a positive bond between parent and child is vital to the child's social adjustment and positive sense of self. The research indicates that a consistent adult model of sharing, helping, comforting, and responsiveness is critical to the young child's development of empathy, moral standards, and self-esteem.[8] Thus, we would expect children who have been abused or neglected to display difficulties in socioemotional arenas. Indeed, nearly every study of the social and emotional development of abused or neglected young children has found evidence of such difficulties, including withdrawal, aggression, noncompliance, poor impulse control, frustration, insensitivity to social situations, lack of empathy, and poor peer relationships.[9]

The well-documented socioemotional difficulties of younger abused or neglected children suggest that older maltreated children might display similar difficulties. Controlled studies of school-age victims, however, have been sorely lacking. Much of our information about maltreated older children has come to us secondhand, through studies of adolescents with other problems such as delinquency, running away, truancy, and drug/alcohol dependency. For a significant number of troubled adolescents, one factor that consistently emerged in these studies was a history of maltreatment–especially physical abuse.

Because these studies did not begin as research on maltreatment, they are unable to show a direct causal relationship between maltreatment and socioemotional problems; theoretically, however, maltreatment could be a causative factor in such problems. The severe parental shortcomings implied by the terms abuse and neglect would be expected to interfere with the child's mastery of the tasks of normal socioemotional development. For adolescents, these tasks primarily involve issues of identity formation, problem solving, and independence–issues which are central to problems such as delinquency, running away, truancy, and drug/alcohol dependency. We expected that the school-age maltreated children in our study (especially the adolescents) would display these kinds of problems.

There is no similar body of research that can provide even secondhand information on preadolescent maltreated children, probably because the problems of middle childhood are less visible and less disruptive to society. However, child development studies do show that variations in parenting styles during the middle years (ages 6 to 12) are related to certain child characteristics. For example, uninvolved, self-centered parenting at this stage is associated with undercontrolled, impulsive behavior in children; overly directive, authoritarian parenting is associated with aggressive, antisocial child behavior; and physical punishment is associated with low self-esteem in children of this age.[10]

Again, these studies cannot show that the aberrant parenting styles caused the negative child behaviors and characteristics, but theories of child development do support this hypothesis. The developmental tasks of middle childhood revolve around issues of self-control, social competence, and self-concept. Parental inadequacies during these years would likely interfere with the child's mastery of these tasks, thus contributing to the specific kinds of behavioral, interpersonal, and self-esteem problems that were identified in the child development studies. By inference, serious abuse or neglect (representing extreme parental inadequacies) could lead to severe difficulties along these same dimensions of development.

Because maltreated children are almost always studied only after maltreatment has occurred, it could be argued (and has been) that those who have been studied may have started out with "difficult temperaments" or constitutional defects which made them both more vulnerable to maltreatment and more likely to score poorly on various measures. If this were true, maltreatment could not be said to have "caused" the children's academic and socioemotional difficulties–these children were simply born different.

However, the ongoing longitudinal research of Egeland and his associates clearly suggests that this is not the case.[11] They found no differences in the dispositions, responsiveness, or other developmental characteristics of infants who were later either maltreated or not maltreated. Only in the second year of life, after some of the children had been maltreated, did differences emerge. The maltreated children functioned much more poorly than comparison children at each subsequent stage of development. At last report, the maltreated children were displaying severe academic and socioemotional problems in kindergarten.[12]

Common sense might suggest that the socioemotional effects of maltreatment would be different for abused and neglected children: that abused children would show more aggression while neglected children would be more withdrawn. However, numerous studies have established that similar outcomes may be expected for both abused and neglected young children,[13] and other studies have found high numbers of both abused and neglected adolescents among delinquent populations.[14] Developmental theories suggest that parental inadequacies in either direction (overcontrolling or underinvolved) affect children of the same developmental stage similarly because both extremes interfere with mastery of the specific tasks of that stage.

Adaptive Functioning

The practical adaptation by abused or neglected children to their environments has never been systematically examined, even for younger maltreated children. It might seem that the child of an abusive or neglectful family would manage to learn behaviors with adaptive or survival value, such as self-care and domestic skills, motor skills, and finding one's way around the community. Child development research suggests, however, that parental shortcomings hinder the development of such behaviors in children. Cognitive stimulation, consistent care, and available reinforcement are fundamental to the development of autonomy, initiative, and industry.[15] Both overly punitive and overly permissive parenting styles have been linked to delays in children's competence and responsibility.[16] By analogy, we expected the abused or neglected children in our study to score below their same-age peers on measures of practical skills.

MALTREATMENT HISTORY

We primarily wanted to determine how the abused or neglected children differed from their nonmaltreated peers, but we were also interested in how maltreated children differed from each other as a result of specific maltreatment histories. It would seem that more severe, chronic, or multiform (e.g., combinations of physical abuse, neglect, sexual abuse) maltreatment would lead to more serious developmental problems, but researchers have rarely examined these factors. Thus, it was primarily on intuitive grounds that we expected to find more serious outcomes for children who had experienced more severe or chronic maltreatment, or those who had been victims of more than one type of maltreatment.

Studies on the effects of foster care have presented conflicting evidence: some studies have found better outcomes for children who were placed in foster care; others have found advantages for children who remained at home.[17] In light of the contradictory findings, we hypothesized that no differences would be apparent on our outcome measures as a result of the child's foster care history.

MALTREATING FAMILIES

In contrast with the limited body of research on maltreatment specifics, the literature on abusive and neglectful families is extensive (though few studies have specifically examined the family backgrounds of school-age maltreated children). The factors most consistently linked with maltreating families are low socioeconomic status (SES), stress, parental depression, and social isolation. We expected these factors to characterize the abusive and neglectful families in our study.

SES

Most families identified by authorities as physically abusive or neglectful come from the lower classes. According to the National Center on Child Abuse and Neglect, children from families whose 1986 income was less than $15,000 were seven times more likely to experience maltreatment than children from families with higher incomes.[18] Indeed, the association is so strong that no serious researcher would think of studying maltreatment without controlling for the effects of SES in some manner. Without such controls there is no way to separate the unique effects of maltreatment from the overlapping effects of low SES.

A substantial body of research has documented that low family SES exerts a profound negative influence on virtually every aspect of school-age children's achievement and adjustment.[19] These difficulties are thought to relate to the power-assertive parenting styles, low rates of family interaction, and high levels of stress that are consistently found in low SES families–factors that also play a role in maltreatment.

Stress

Family stress has been implicated in child maltreatment incidents (especially physical abuse) since studies on the topic began. Single parenthood, large family size, unemployment, stressful life events, alcohol and drug problems, and marital conflict have all been linked with maltreatment.[20] Such stressors, especially as they accumulate, increase the likelihood of dysfunctional parent-child relationships.[21]

Parental Depression

The literature on depression provides strong evidence that depressed mothers display both low levels of emotional involvement with and high levels of resentment and hostility toward their children.[22] Thus, it is not surprising that maternal depression has been associated with child abuse and neglect (fathers in maltreating families have rarely been studied).[23]

Social Isolation

Social support, which could serve as a buffer to environmental stressors, may be unavailable to or underutilized by maltreating families. In the 1970s, social isolation was thought to be a primary ingredient in child abuse cases.[24] More recent studies have presented evidence that the lack of social support may not be an important factor in physical abuse,[25] but the links between child neglect and social isolation are well established.[26]

SUMMARY

Previous studies examining the impact of abuse or neglect on children have largely focused on maltreated infants, toddlers, or preschool children. In reality, older children are at greater risk of maltreatment, but well-controlled studies of older abused or neglected children have been sorely lacking. This book describes the first comprehensive effort to examine the specific developmental consequences of maltreatment for the school-age child.

In Chapter One, we explored the realities of child abuse and neglect, identified a range of research questions concerning the older maltreated child, and presented sundry hypotheses based on previous research and theory. In the next chapter, we will describe (using a minimum of jargon) how we conducted the research.

NOTES

1. National Center on Child Abuse and Neglect, *Study Findings. Study of National Incidence and Prevalence of Child Abuse and Neglect: 1988* (Washington, DC: U.S. Government Printing Office, 1988).

2. C.J. Garbarino, C.J. Schellenbach, and I.M. Sebes, *Troubled Youth, Troubled Families: Understanding Families At-Risk for Adolescent Maltreatment* (New York: de Gruyter, 1986).

3. National Center on Child Abuse and Neglect, *Study Findings.*

4. Ibid.

5. F.P. Hughes, L.D. Noppe, and I.C. Noppe, *Child Development* (Los Angeles: West Publishing Co., 1988), 253.

6. R.M. Barahal, J. Waterman, and H.P. Martin, "The Social Cognitive Development of Abused Children," *Journal of Consulting and Clinical Psychology* 49 (1981): 508-16; D. Hoffman-Plotkin and C.T. Twentyman, "A Multimodal Assessment of Behavioral and Cognitive Deficits in Abused and Neglected Preschoolers," *Child Development* 55 (1984): 794-802.

7. Hughes, *Child Development,* 246-54.

8. M.R. Yarrow, P.M. Scott, and C. Waxler, "Learning Concern for Others," *Developmental Psychology* 8 (1973): 240-60; M.L. Hoffman, "Moral Development," in *Carmichael's Manual of Child Psychology,* 2nd ed., ed. P.H. Mussen (New York: Wiley, 1970), 261-359; S. Coopersmith, *The Antecedents of Self-Esteem* (San Francisco: Freeman, 1967).

9. Barahal, "Social Cognitive Development"; Hoffman-Plotkin, "Behavioral and Cognitive Deficits"; B. Egeland, A. Sroufe, and M. Erickson, "The Developmental Consequences of Different Patterns of Maltreatment," *Child Abuse and Neglect* 7 (1983): 459-69; C. George and M. Main, "Social Interactions of Young Abused Children: Approach, Avoidance, and Aggression," *Child Development* 50 (1979): 306-38; G. Straker and R.S. Jacobson, "Aggression, Emotional Maladjustment, and Empathy in the Abused Child," *Developmental Psychology* 17 (1981): 762-5.

10. E.E. Maccoby, "Middle Childhood in the Context of the Family," in *Development During Middle Childhood: The Years from Six to Twelve,* ed. W.A. Collins (Washington, DC: National Academy Press, 1984): 185-239.

11. Egeland, "Developmental Consequences."

12. M.F. Erickson, B. Egeland, and R. Pianta, "The Effects of Maltreatment on the Development of Young Children," in *Child Maltreatment: Theory and Research on the Causes and Consequences of Child Abuse and Neglect,* ed. D. Cicchetti and V. Carlson (New York: Cambridge University Press, 1989), 647-84.

13. Straker, "Aggression"; D.M. Bousha and C.T. Twentyman, "Mother-Child Interactional Style in Abuse, Neglect, and Control Groups: Naturalistic Observations in the Home," *Journal of Abnormal Psychology* 93 (1984): 106-14.

14. J.D. Alfaro, "Report on the Relationship between Child Abuse and Neglect and Later Socially Deviant Behavior," in *Exploring the Relationship between Child Abuse and Delinquency,* ed. R.J. Hanner and Y.E. Walker (Montclair, NJ: Allanheld, Osmun, and Co., 1981): 175-219; S.E. Brown, "Social Class, Child Maltreatment, and Delinquent Behavior," *Criminology* 22 (1984): 259-78; C.P. Smith, D.J. Berkman, and W.M. Fraser, *A Preliminary National Assessment of Child Abuse and Neglect and the Juvenile Justice System: The Shadow of Distress* (Washington, DC: U.S. Department of Justice, Office of Juvenile Justice and Delinquency Prevention, 1980).

15. E.H. Erikson, *Childhood and Society,* 2nd ed. (New York: W. W. Norton, 1963).

16. D. Baumrind, "Authoritarian vs. Authoritative Parental Control," *Adolescence* 3 (1968): 255-72; D. Baumrind, "Current Patterns of Parental Authority," *Developmental Psychology Monographs* 4 (1971): 99-103.

17. D. Fanshel and E.B. Shinn, *Children in Foster Care: A Longitudinal Investigation* (New York: Columbia University Press, 1978); J.T. Kent, "A Follow-Up Study of Abused Children," *Journal of Pediatric Psychology* 1 (1976): 25-31; M.A. Lynch and J. Roberts, *Consequences of Child Abuse* (London: Academic Press, 1982); E. Elmer, *Fragile Families, Troubled Children: The Aftermath of Infant Trauma* (Pittsburgh: University of Pittsburgh Press, 1977).

18. National Center on Child Abuse and Neglect, *Study Findings.*

19. K.S. Berger, *The Developing Person Through Childhood and Adolescence,* 2nd ed. (New York: Worth, 1986): 441-2.

20. M. Morris and R. Gould, *The Neglected Battered Child Syndrome* (New York: Child Welfare League of America, 1975); I. Wolock and B. Horowitz, "Child Maltreatment and Maternal Deprivation Among AFDC-Recipient Families," *Social Service Review* 53 (1979): 530-43; L.D. Steinberg, R. Catalano, and D. Dooley, "Economic Antecedents of Child Abuse and Neglect," *Child Development* 52 (1981): 975-85; R.L. Burgess and R.D. Conger, "Family Interaction Patterns Related to Child Abuse and Neglect: Some Preliminary Findings," *Child Abuse and Neglect* 1 (1977): 269-77; D.A. Wolfe, P. Jaffe, S.K. Wilson, and L. Zak, "Children of Battered Women: The Relation of Child Behavior to Family Violence and Maternal Stress," *Journal of Consulting and Clinical Psychology* 53 (1985): 657-65.

21. Maccoby, "Middle Childhood," 210.

22. M.M. Weissman and E.S. Paykel, *The Depressed Woman: A Study of Social Relationships* (Chicago: University of Chicago Press, 1974); D. Belle, ed., *Lives in Stress: Women and Depression* (Beverly Hills: Sage, 1982).

23. B.B. Lahey, R.D. Conger, B.M. Atkinson, and F.A. Treiber, "Parenting Behavior and Emotional Status of Physically Abusive Mothers," *Journal of Consulting and Clinical Psychology* 52 (1984): 1062-71; C. Webster-Stratton, "Comparison of Abusive and Nonabusive Families with Conduct-Disordered Children," *American Journal of Orthopsychiatry* 55, no. 1 (1985): 59-69; N.A. Polanski, C. Hally, and N.F. Polanski, *Profile of Neglect–A Survey of the State of the Knowledge of Child Neglect* (Washington, DC: U.S. Department of Education and Welfare, Community Services Administration, 1975).

24. J. Garbarino, "The Human Ecology of Maltreatment: A Conceptual Model for Research," *Journal of Marriage and the Family* 39 (1977): 721-36.

25. E.A.W. Seagull, "Social Support and Child Maltreatment: A Review of the Evidence," *Child Abuse and Neglect* 11 (1987): 41-52.

26. N.A. Polanski, M.A. Chalmers, C. Buttenweiser, and D. P. Williams, "Isolation of the Neglectful Family," *American Journal of Orthopsychiatry* 49 (1979): 149-52; J.M. Giovanni and A. Billingsley, "Child Neglect Among the Poor: A Study of Parental Adequacy in Families of Three Ethnic Groups," *Child Welfare* 49 (1970): 196-206.

Chapter Two

Research in Action

Studying child abuse is no easy matter. For ethical reasons, the classic experimental approach cannot be used. We cannot randomly assign babies to abusive or nonabusive parents, nor can we subject children to abusive punishment or deprivation in the laboratory (this has been done with dogs, rhesus monkeys, and other unlucky laboratory animals). Instead, we must design field studies around children who have been maltreated in their real-world settings.

Field studies that are poorly conducted are useless or misleading, and even the best field studies cannot establish a direct cause-effect relationship between maltreatment and children's poor functioning. Good field research, however, can provide rich evidence for making causal inferences. Furthermore, the inherent weaknesses of field research can be partially overcome by sound methodology.

We set out to strengthen our study by adhering to established principles of research design and procedure. These rules of the game are based on abstract principles of logic, but what they really come down to is common sense. It is obvious that studying one abused child will not tell you very much about abused children; studying 100 abused children will not tell you much either unless you compare these children with others who have not been abused but who have similar backgrounds in other ways. Likewise, relying on only one questionnaire or one source of information weakens the usefulness of a study, especially if the questionnaire is defective or the source is biased (as an abusive parent might be). Further, studies that examine children at only one point in time are unable to distinguish between transient and more enduring effects of maltreatment.

Given the resources at our disposal, these methodological problems were easily avoided: we designed the study to include an appropriate comparison group, multiple measuring instruments of demonstrated validity, multiple sources of information, and follow-up interviews. These and other principles of research were built in at the design stage. However, field research is hardly static, and efforts to strengthen studies are frequently compromised by the realities of the real world. Human systems and individuals do not always operate the way we expect they will; the information we seek is not always found where we expect it to be; the best laid plans can go awry in a thousand and one ways. A sound research design helps, but the credibility of a study hangs on the ability and resourcefulness of the researchers as they apply creative problem-solving strategies day by day.

This chapter describes the study's methodology–the who, what, when, where, how, and why of each aspect of measurement, site selection, participant selection, information collection, and data analysis.

MEASUREMENT

During the design stage, our careful review of prior research and established theories led to the formulation of numerous hypotheses. We then had to determine how to measure the concepts specified in these hypotheses. First, each concept had to be converted into a variable (something numerically measurable) that could show whether a child or family scored high or low on that concept. For example, the concept of school performance was converted into such variables as language skills, math skills, and grade repeats. With this information we would be able to compare the children on specific aspects of their academic progress and compute an overall score for each child that would reflect school performance.

Next, we had to determine some way of measuring each variable that would be considered valid (i.e., accurate, adequate, conceptually sound). Since test construction and validation is a science in itself, we searched the literature in an effort to locate existing instruments that could measure the variables we had identified. We were especially concerned that the instruments reflect the specific developmental issues of school-age children. We also considered instrument suitability for use with low SES/low functioning children or adults.

We were able to locate a number of excellent instruments suitable for our purposes, though a few had to be modified or shortened. For some variables, however, appropriate instruments were not available, and we had to construct our own the best we could. In these cases, while the instruments we devised do appear to measure what they were intended to measure (i.e., have face validity), they were not formally validated. All instruments were pilot tested before the actual study began, and all were judged able to provide usable and reasonably sound information.

Measures Used

To measure school performance, we collected the following information: (1) test scores on the language and math portions of the IOWA Test of Basic Skills (a standardized test used in every state); (2) reading and math scores from the Georgia Criterion Reference Test (a test of basic academic skills administered statewide); (3) grades in language and math; (4) teacher assessments of the child's classroom performance; (5) grade repeats; and (6) absences.

The concept of socioemotional development was broken down into nine variables:

1. problem behaviors as assessed by a parent,
2. problem behaviors as assessed by a teacher,
3. self-concept,
4. aggression,
5. emotional adjustment,
6. home adjustment,
7. school adjustment,
8. peer relationships,
9. delinquency.

Problem behaviors were measured using the parent and teacher forms of the Child Behavior Checklist, which is undoubtedly the most widely used and well-validated instrument available for measuring the problem behaviors of school age children.[1] Self-concept was assessed through the Piers-Harris Children's Self-Concept Scale, also highly regarded and extensively validated for children of this age.[2] The Jesness Inventory (Manifest Aggression Subscale) was used to measure aggression. This measure is used less often and, while it is not as fully validated as the prior instruments, it is probably the best instrument available for detecting school-age children's feelings of anger and hostility.[3]

The child's school adjustment, home adjustment, emotional adjustment, peer relationships, and delinquency were assessed, in part, through questions from the Child Assessment Schedule. While this measure is a recent addition to the field, it is already supported by impressive validity reports.[4] Measures for these variables also included questions from other instruments, including the Child Behavior Checklist, the Piers-Harris, and a parent interview constructed by the researchers.

The concept of adaptive functioning was assessed using three scales from the Woodcock-Johnson Scales of Independent Behavior, which has been extensively used and validated, especially with institutionalized and handicapped children and adults.[5] We used the scales that measure the variables of motor development (gross motor skills and fine motor skills), personal care skills (eating, toileting, dressing, self-care, and domestic skills), and community skills (time and punctuality, money and value, work skills, and home-community orientation). Table 1 shows sample items from the socioemotional and adaptive functioning measures used.

Information about maltreatment specifics (i.e., severity, chronicity, multiple forms of maltreatment, sexual abuse, foster care) was obtained from caseworkers based on their knowledge and the child's CPS record. The caseworker form included 19 scales from the Child Well-Being Scales, a fairly well-validated instrument designed to measure the unmet needs of children in maltreatment situations.[6] These scales were used to measure the severity of neglect for all maltreating families. Three scales from the same instrument were used as a rudimentary measure of neglect for all families (maltreating and nonmaltreating) who participated in the study. This was to serve as verification of the presence of neglect in neglectful families and its absence in comparison families.

Similarly, both maltreating and nonmaltreating families were administered the Conflict Tactics Scale to assess the extent of verbal and physical aggression between parents and children.[7] This instrument is the most widely used and well-validated measure currently available for research on family violence, although a number of reports suggest that perpetrators of violence may seriously underreport their use of aggressive tactics when responding to the questions from this instrument.[8]

SES levels were computed for each family based on income, parent education, parent occupation, quality of housing, and quality of neighborhood. For abused or neglected children in foster care, SES scores were adjusted downward to reflect the SES means of their respective groups. This was done to avoid misrepresentation of the temporary advantages some children might obtain through foster care placement. The adjustment would, if anything, make it harder to show differences among the groups on outcome measures. Thus, it did not pose a threat to the study's integrity.

The concept of family stress was measured in a variety of ways. Information about single parenthood, unemployment, family size, and marital conflict was assessed through questions asked of parents and children. We measured stressful life events using the Life Events Inventory, which calculates the impact of stressful events on families over the past year.[9] Although this instrument has not been fully validated, there is evidence that it is a reliable gauge of family stress levels.

Since we were unable to locate appropriate instruments for measuring parent depression and social isolation, we constructed our own questions to assess these variables. For parent depression, we asked the responding parent four questions regarding his or her general emotional state. Social support was assessed through parent responses to seven questions dealing with the availability and use of instrumental support from relatives, friends, neighbors, and community resources; the frequency of visits with relatives and friends; and the frequency of church attendance. Table 2 gives sample items from family measures used.

We knew that some of the maltreated children in our study would be in foster care and that we would have to interview a foster parent rather than a natural or step-parent in these cases. As it turned out, three (13%) abused and nine (19%) neglected children were in foster care at the time of the initial interviews, and six (27%) abused and nine (19%) neglected children were in foster or institutional care at follow-up. In these cases, all information provided by the

TABLE 1. Sample Items from Socioemotional Measures

Measure	Sample Items	Responses	Asked Of
Problem behavior (112 items)	Argues a lot Gets in many fights Shy or timid Threatens people	Not true; somewhat true; very true	Teacher; parent
Self-concept (80 items)	I am a happy person. I am popular. I often get into trouble.	Yes; no	Child
Aggression (31 items)	I have very strange and funny thoughts in my mind. When I get really mad, I'll do just about anything. When somebody orders me to do something, I usually feel like doing just the opposite.	True; false	Child
School adjustment (24 items)	How far do you think you [he/she] will go in school?	[grade levels; years of post high school]	Child; parent
	Compared to typical students of the same age, this child is happy...	Much less; somewhat less; about average; somewhat; much more	Teacher
	Do you have more trouble than most kids in following rules at school?	Yes; no; uncertain	Child

Home adjustment (9 items)	How do you get along with your mother?	Well; so so; poorly	Child
	Do you wish there was anything different about your family?	More material goods; family member's behavior; self; family composition; other	Child
	Has he/she ever run away from home?	Yes; no	Parent
Emotional adjustment (22 items)	Do you ever feel like bad or terrible things will happen to you?	Yes; no; uncertain	Child
	How often do you have trouble falling asleep?	Once a week or more; once every few weeks; seldom or never	Child
	Has [name] ever attempted or seriously talked about suicide?	Yes; no	Parent
Peer relationships (10 items)	How old are your best friends?	Within 2 years; younger; older	Child
	What do you like to do with friends?	Reports activities; cannot report activities	Child
	How does he/she get along with other kids?	Very well; fairly well so so; poorly; very poorly	Parent
Delinquency (20 items)	Were you [was he/she] ever arrested or sent to juvenile court?	Yes; no; uncertain	Child; parent
	Have you ever...set a fire?	Yes; no	Child
	Has he/she [have you] ever drunk alcohol or used drugs a lot or too much?	Yes; no	Parent; child

Note. Problem behavior = Child Behavior Checklist; self concept = Piers-Harris Children's Self-Concept Scale; aggression = Jesness Manifest Aggression Subscale; school adjustment, home adjustment, emotional adjustment, peer relationships, delinquency = some items adapted from Child Assessment Schedule.

TABLE 2. Sample Items from Family Measures

Measure	Sample Items	Responses
Stressful life events (48 items)	Trouble with superiors at work Immediate family member starts drinking heavily Unwanted pregnancy	[circle events that occured in past year]
Social support (9 items)	How many [...relatives] do you regularly receive help from when needed (e.g., babysitting)? How many times did you visit with [...friends] (at your home or theirs) in the past month? How many times did you attend religious services in the past month?	[number]
Parental depression (4 items)	I consider myself a happy person. I expect some interesting and pleasant things to happen to me. I feel there is more disappointment in life than satisfaction.	Strongly agree; agree; unsure; disagree; strongly disagree

Note. Stressful life events = Life Events Inventory.

foster parent (or house parent) regarding the child's functioning was used in the data analyses, but information on the foster parent's stress, depression, social isolation, physical aggression, and interviewer rating of neglect were not. Inclusion of this information would only have muddied the waters because we were trying to establish a connection between these factors and maltreatment. It may seem useless to collect information that is not to be used, but the section on information collection later in this chapter will explain why it was important for foster families to be treated exactly the same way as natural families.

SITE SELECTION

Our research was to depend upon the cooperation of CPS (Child Protective Services) agencies and school systems. We were asking caseworkers and teachers to take time out of their busy schedules to fill out our forms and (for caseworkers) to contact prospective participants; we were asking supervisors to identify eligible participants, collect forms, and coordinate efforts; and we were asking CPS directors and school superintendents to consent to this intrusion on their workers' time. In addition, we were asking for guarantees that confidentiality would be strictly maintained. For CPS, this meant that caseworkers could not let parents, foster parents, or others know the real purpose of the study. For school systems, it meant that teachers, principals, office secretaries, and other in-school personnel could not be advised as to the nature of the study or the inclusion of maltreated children.

The state of Georgia contains 159 counties, each with its own CPS office and independent school system. Obviously, we had not planned to study all school-age abused or neglected children from all these counties; we had to select a small number of counties to work with. We would need between five and ten counties to participate in order to obtain a sample of sufficient size to run all the statistical tests we had in mind. These counties would have to represent different geographical regions of Georgia and include rural, small town, suburban, and urban settings. We identified about 20 suitable sites because we knew that a number of systems would decline to participate.

We first contacted state and regional CPS directors, explained what we wanted to do, and asked for general approval of the project. Once this was granted, we approached community CPS directors and school administrators in each selected county with our proposal. This process began with an introductory telephone call, which was followed by a mailing of detailed information on the study and, when these efforts brought positive responses, a visit to the prospective site.

We met with directors, superintendents, supervisors, caseworkers, school social workers, and other system personnel throughout Georgia to talk about the project. We explained the importance of our mission and what we wanted from them. In most cases, we were warmly received. More than a few systems seemed to feel honored to be included, despite the burdensome tasks we were asking them to take on. Others were justifiably concerned about such a heavy commitment and left it up to caseworkers, committees, or boards to decide. For a county to be included in the study, both CPS and the school system had to agree to cooperate. In a few counties, one or the other was disappointed (as were we) that their counterpart declined to participate.

Through our initial efforts, we were able to secure seven geographically and demographically diverse counties as study sites. As the study began, however, it became apparent that CPS offices in the participating counties were having difficulty providing a sufficient number of maltreatment cases. We decided to resume the cumbersome process of identifying, contacting, and visiting additional sites. In the end, we added two more counties to our roster, for a total of nine.

PARTICIPANT SELECTION

The question of who is to be compared with whom is crucial to a study's credibility. Ideally, the maltreated children in our study were to be clear-cut abuse or neglect cases and to be representative of all school-age children in Georgia who had been abused or neglected. The comparison children's histories would be identical to those of the maltreated children except that they had never been maltreated. Realistically, these ideal conditions would be nearly impossible to attain. In field studies, ideal principles of research regarding participant selection inevitably collide with practical considerations.

The Maltreatment Groups

Almost all maltreatment researchers rely on CPS to provide maltreated participants, as we did. Unfortunately, there are several problems with this method. In our case, it meant that CPS investigators and caseworkers would be defining our sample, and they might not do this in a very scientific manner. Both reporting and case substantiation decisions are subject to various sorts of bias. A child might be considered abused by one worker but not by another; abused in one county but neglected in the next. As a result, there might be some overlap between our "abused" and "neglected" groups, and our groups might not be representative of all abuse or neglect cases.

We were aware of these problems, of course, and did what we could to minimize their impact on the study. We built in several checks on CPS classifications by collecting specific information about each child far beyond the classification of abuse or neglect–information about the severity, chronicity, characteristics, extent, and forms of the abuse or neglect. We also gathered information from other sources: interviewers rated each family's home environment on three scales of neglect, and all parents were asked about their use of aggressive conflict tactics in the home. (As it turned out, our results supported the validity of caseworker classifications.)

We also had to depend on CPS workers in another crucial way. Our study design required the informed consent of participating parents who could choose to participate only after the procedures and risks were explained to them. They had to be informed that the information obtained would not be released in any individually identifiable form unless required by law, and that evidence of ongoing abuse or neglect would have to be reported. We would not be able to obtain this consent ourselves from CPS parents. Legally, we had no access to these parents, whose confidentiality was guaranteed by law. It was up to caseworkers to approach the parents, invite them to participate, and obtain signatures on consent forms. This situation presents a nightmare for researchers, who aim to control every aspect of their study.

To reduce any threat to the study's integrity, we provided training, sample scripts, and payment ($20 per case obtained, plus mileage) to caseworkers. They were instructed to present the project as a study of child development and school performance. Parents were promised $10 for each of two interviews if they and their children participated (children would receive $5 for each interview). In foster cases, a CPS supervisor could sign the consent because CPS had custody of these children, and foster parents were invited to participate in the same way as natural parents, receiving the same reimbursement.

Children in foster care could participate only if they had been in the same placement for at least three months (so foster parents would know the child well enough to answer our questions). Other criteria for determining participation eligibility were also stipulated. All children were to be 8 to 16 years of age and could display no evidence of severe neurological impairment such as autism. The child's primary classification had to be physical abuse or neglect, and the most recent substantiated report of abuse or neglect must have occurred within the previous 18 months. Only one child per family could participate.

We knew that caseworkers' approach to parents would vary, that they might hesitate to approach parents who were hostile toward CPS, and that some parents might decline to participate for various reasons. These factors could lead to a biased sample because parents who were not approached or who declined to participate might differ from participants in important ways that might affect our results. However, with all that we were asking of caseworkers, we were reluctant to ask them to keep a record of all parent contacts. We doubted that we would receive accurate accounts at any rate. We suspected abusive parents would be more likely than neglectful parents to view CPS workers and researchers with hostility. We also thought abusive parents might be less likely to be approached by caseworkers or to agree to participate in the study if they were approached.

Thus, when referrals started coming in and it became apparent that neglect cases were outnumbering abuse cases two to one, we became concerned that these kinds of selection biases were occurring frequently. However, a check of on-site records revealed that referrals were proportional to eligible cases of abuse and neglect. The records showed that neglect cases were twice as common as abuse cases in participating counties (this ratio is also reflected in national statistics). Further, most substantiated abuse cases involved children younger than those we wanted to study. This was not true of neglect cases, perhaps because all children in a neglectful family may be classified as neglected whereas abuse is more likely to involve only one child. Thus, while some abusive parents may not have been approached or may have declined to participate, this was apparently not a frequent occurrence. At any rate, in both these instances, nonparticipation would likely reflect more serious abuse or other pathology. Therefore, the loss to the study would result in underestimation rather than exaggeration of any academic, socioemotional, or functional delays found in physically abused children.

At the conclusion of the participant selection process, a total of 22 physically abused and 47 neglected children (and their families) formed our maltreatment groups. These numbers were deemed adequate for the statistical procedures we planned to conduct.

The Comparison Group

In order to make causal inferences from our study results, a comparison group had to be assembled that was similar to the maltreatment groups except for the maltreatment. Our first consideration involved how to control for SES. Many studies that use a comparison group select only low SES children and their families as comparison group participants. This approach is methodologically sound and permits causal inferences to be drawn from the study's findings. However, by limiting the scope of possible comparisons, it does not allow a complete profile of the abused or neglected child to emerge. We wanted to know how maltreated children and their families stacked up against a broad sample of typical children and families.

To make this wider range of comparison possible while still allowing us to disentangle the effects of maltreatment from the effects of poverty and class, we elected to use established statistical procedures to control for SES (see the section on data analysis in this chapter). This method provides a rich foundation for understanding the developmental consequences and family characteristics of abuse or neglect in the context of larger societal norms and conditions.

To ensure similarity between the comparison children and the maltreated children in terms of age, sex, race, locality, etc., we selected comparison children from the same schools and classes the maltreated children were attending. First, school administrators and social workers helped us randomly select classes from various grade levels (we drew numbers from a hat). All children from the selected classes took home letters inviting parents and children to participate in the study. The letters described the project in the same way caseworkers had described it to maltreatment parents (as a study of child development and school performance), and the same level of reimbursement was offered for each interview ($10 for parents; $5 for children).

Families who were interested in participating returned a form. From these, we selected participants in a semi-random fashion, balancing age, sex, race, and residence factors. We then contacted selected parents to explain the procedures we would use and to obtain informed consent. The names of prospective comparison participants were forwarded to CPS administrators who checked their files to verify that the children had no history of reported maltreatment. One child who did was dropped from the comparison group.

INFORMATION COLLECTION

Information was collected in a variety of ways. After caseworkers obtained signed consent forms from parents, the caseworkers filled out questionnaires about each identified child and family. School administrators arranged for teachers to fill out the Child Behavior Checklist about each participating child. Most of the information we needed, however, had to be obtained through interviews set up with parents and children. Thus, for each locality we had to find an experienced interviewer who was willing and able to travel and work flexible hours, including evenings and Saturdays when necessary.

As soon as our initial sites were selected, we placed ads in the local newspapers to solicit résumés from qualified individuals in each county. Responses began to pour in, and interviews were scheduled with the best qualified candidates. In the end, eight interviewers were hired. All had attained at least master's degrees in the social sciences, were experienced interviewers, and were deemed able to establish rapport with children and adults of varied backgrounds.

One of the most important considerations when collecting research information is to reduce possible sources of bias. Bias usually reflects a distortion in favor of what is expected. For instance, interviewers who expect abused or neglected children to score below nonmaltreated children on various measures might interpret the children's responses to questions accordingly. This potential problem was overcome by assuring that interviewers were "blind" to the purpose of the study and the inclusion of maltreated children. Thus, for interviewers as well as parents, teachers, children, and on-site school personnel, the project was described as a study of child development and school performance. Furthermore, participants were in no way identified as belonging to different groups; all parents and children were treated in exactly the same manner.

The interviewers received procedural training for arranging the interviews and administering the instruments. Specific directions were given regarding the order in which to administer the instruments and how to code responses, answer questions from participants, and probe for additional information when necessary. Interviewers were also taught how to record information from the child's permanent school record. When training was complete, the interviewers were provided with the same information about all participants–names, addresses, phone numbers, schools, and directions to the home. They were instructed to contact parents and schools and arrange mutually agreed-upon times for the interviews to take place.

The parent interviews, which lasted for approximately an hour and a half, took place in the families' homes. This made it easier for parents logistically and helped to prevent missed appointments. It also allowed interviewers to assess the family's home environment. The children were interviewed at their schools for 30 to 40 minutes. Schools were considered a neutral environment for the children, who might respond with more reserve if they thought parents or other family members could overhear from the next room.

The same information had to be collected about children and parents at follow-up. Thus, during the second year of the project, we again contacted CPS offices and schools to begin the process of tracking down the first-year participants. Some had moved out of state and had to be dropped from the follow-up portion of the study. Others had moved within the state and, in these cases, we made every attempt to include the children and their families in the follow-up. In most of these instances we were able to obtain permission from schools and other institutions to proceed and to arrange for our interviewers to travel to the additional sites. Altogether, 19 abused (86%), 40 neglected (85%), and 60 comparison (86%) children and their families were included at follow-up.

Originally, we planned follow-up interviews to take place 12 months after the initial interviews for all participants. However, as previously mentioned, we decided to augment our sample after it became apparent that we needed more cases for statistical purposes. Because of the resulting lag time in securing additional sites, initial and follow-up interviews did not always take place 12 months apart; in some cases, the interviews were closer to six months apart. This change in our original plan resulted in modifications of the data analysis procedures (described below) we would use for analyzing follow-up information.

Approximately two years after the follow-up interviews took place, we contacted CPS and school personnel once again to request updates on the maltreated children. The information generated was too spotty to subject to statistical analysis, but it will be presented anecdotally in later chapters.

DATA ANALYSIS

Once the first-year information was collected, master's level graduate assistants entered the numerically coded responses into computers according to preplanned coding schemes. The information could then be stored in usable form. Our statistician would be able to systematically order and manipulate the information to provide answers to our research questions. From the output (endless reams of computer printout) we could determine whether expected patterns were actually found.

Our model for data analysis procedures followed from our research design and the specific hypotheses we had proposed. The study involved a great many variables and the complex relationships among them. Accordingly, we used multivariate analysis procedures (Analysis of Covariance) that would allow us to assess the effect of one variable while taking another or several other variables into account.

For example, each family's SES level was statistically adjusted for every outcome variable examined. Thus, the output from the statistical procedures could tell us how scores on each instrument were related to SES and whether there were differences among the groups (abused, neglected, nonmaltreated) after SES differences were "partialed out" or eliminated. The output could also tell us whether the differences were significant, that is, of greater magnitude than differences that might have occurred by chance.

Our data analysis procedures produced surprising results from the very beginning when we discovered an unexpected racial disparity among our groups. According to the latest National Incidence Study, there are no significant racial differences nationwide in reports of any subcategory of maltreatment.[10] Thus, we had not anticipated that 80% of our neglect families would be white while only 55% of the abuse families and 63% of the comparison families where white. Because of this difference, we had to implement statistical controls to examine the separate contribution of race on outcome measures. As will be discussed in the following chapters, there were few significant effects of race, and in only one case (teacher-reported problem behaviors) did our statistical controls for race change the preliminary results of the study. Table A of the Appendix presents raw differences (without controls for SES) among the groups on demographic variables.

To assess differences among the three groups over time, we combined initial and follow-up information and used a repeated measures factorial design, with SES controlled. In order to determine whether the children had improved or lost ground between initial and follow-up interviews, we first split the groups into high and low SES children and families. We then compared the degree of change for each group. This procedure resulted in six groups: 16 low SES abused, 3 high SES abused, 37 low SES neglected, 3 high SES neglected, 19 low SES nonmaltreated, and 41 high SES nonmaltreated children and families. The follow-up results presented in later chapters reflect changes for the low SES groups.

SUMMARY

A field study's credibility depends on the nuts and bolts decisions that are made regarding each aspect of measurement, site selection, participant selection, information collection, and data analysis. This chapter detailed the problems that confront child abuse and neglect researchers, and it explained how such problems were dealt with in The University of Georgia Child Maltreatment Project. Answering the research questions posed in Chapter One required a massive outlay of time, effort, and resources. In the end, we were confident that our diligence had established a sound foundation for discerning the consequences of abuse and neglect for the school-age child. Now we were ready to take a look at the results. These are presented in Chapters Three through Six.

NOTES

1. T.M. Achenbach and C.S. Edelbrock, *Child Behavior Checklist* (Burlington, VT: University of Vermont, Center for Children, Youth, and Families, 1980).
2. E.V. Piers, *Piers-Harris Children's Self-Concept Scale: Revised Manual 1984* (Los Angeles: Western Psychological Services, 1986).
3. C.F. Jesness, *Manual: The Jesness Inventory* (Palo Alto, CA: Consulting Psychologists Press, 1983).
4. K. Hodges, "Assessing Children with a Clinical Research Interview: The Child Assessment Schedule," *Advances in Behavioral Assessment of Children and Families* 3 (1987): 203-33.
5. R.H. Bruininks, R.W. Woodcock, R.F. Weatherman, and B.K. Hill, *Scales of Independent Behavior: Woodcock-Johnson Psycho-Educational Battery, Part IV* (Allen, TX: DLM Teacher Resources, 1984).
6. S. Magura and B.S. Moses, *Outcome Measures for Child Welfare Services: Theory and Application* (Washington, DC: Child Welfare League of America, 1986).

7. M.A. Straus, "Measuring Intrafamily Conflict and Violence: The Conflict Tactics (CT) Scales," *Journal of Marriage and the Family* 41 (1979): 75-88.

8. M.A. Straus, "The Conflict Tactics Scales: An Evaluation and New Data on Validity, Reliability, Norms, and Scoring Methods," (paper presented at the National Council on Family Relations, Durham, NH, October, 1987).

9. R. Cochrane and A. Robertson, "The Life Events Inventory: A Measure of the Relative Severity of Psycho-Social Stressors," *Journal of Psychosomatic Research* 17 (1973): 135-9.

10. National Center on Child Abuse and Neglect, *Study Findings. Study of National Incidence and Prevalence of Child Abuse and Neglect: 1988* (Washington, DC: U.S. Government Printing Office, 1988).

Chapter Three

Overview of Findings

The massive amount of information we collected on school-age maltreated children produced an extensive array of findings which cannot be easily summarized. The results of our study did provide substantial evidence of the negative and lasting consequences of maltreatment for school-age children. As expected, the maltreating families reported experiencing far more life difficulties than nonmaltreating families. In several respects, the problems of the maltreated children and their families were far more severe than we had imagined, but we also found distinct strengths where we had not expected to find them. A number of our hypotheses about important variables were simply not supported by the data.

EFFECTS OF PHYSICAL ABUSE

The physically abused children experienced an overwhelming set of problems in school, at home, among peers, and in the community. They differed significantly from comparison children on all ten of our basic measures of academic and socioemotional development (see Figures 1-14; Tables B and C, Appendix). The abused children's difficulties were particularly apparent on measures of school performance, problem behavior in the home, aggression, adjustment problems in school and with peers, and delinquency. At follow-up, the children's problems had improved slightly on most measures, but problems with school performance and behavior had increased (see Table D, Appendix).

Without effective intervention, these children are likely to experience continuing and severe dysfunction. Indeed, by the time the

FIGURE 1. School Performance: Language

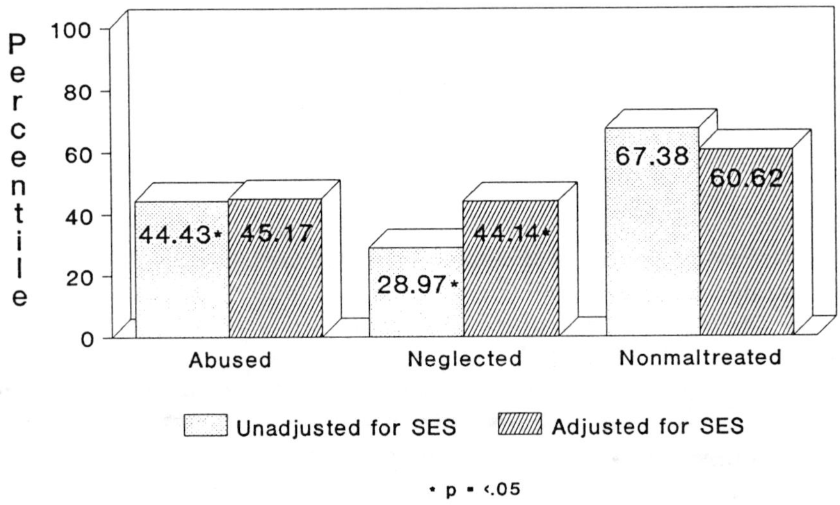

FIGURE 2. School Performance: Math

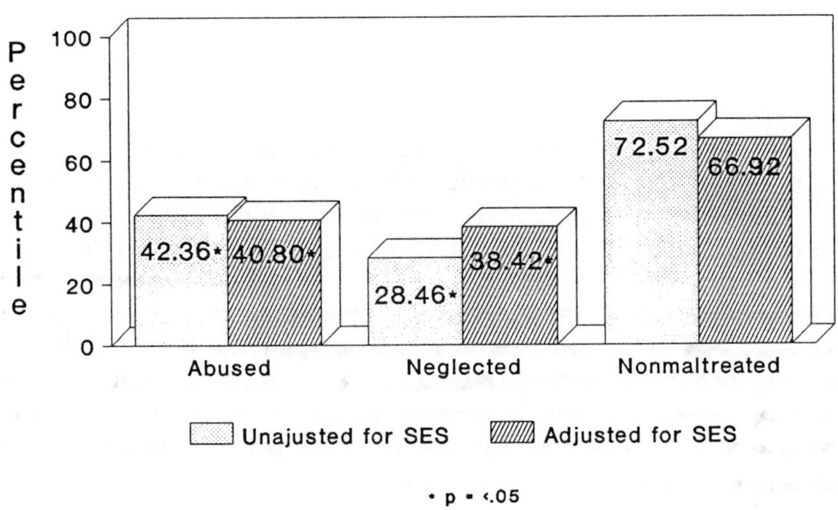

FIGURE 3. School Performance: Grade Repeats

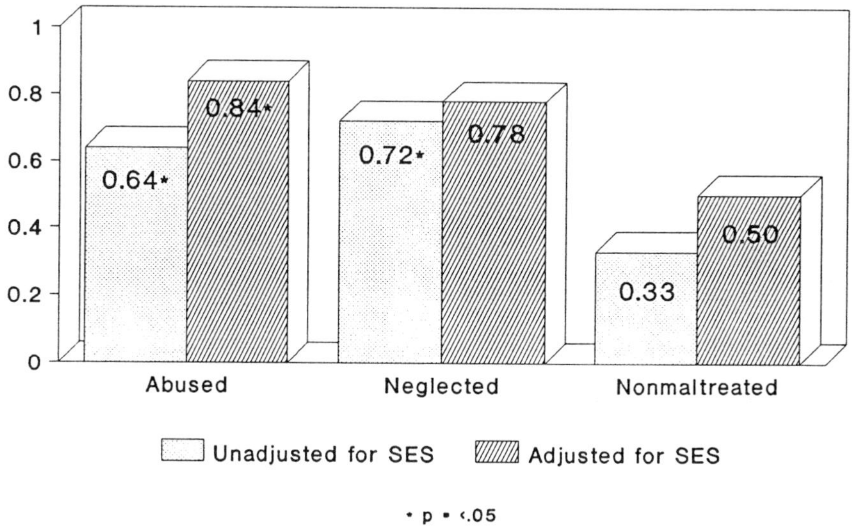

FIGURE 4. School Performance: Absences

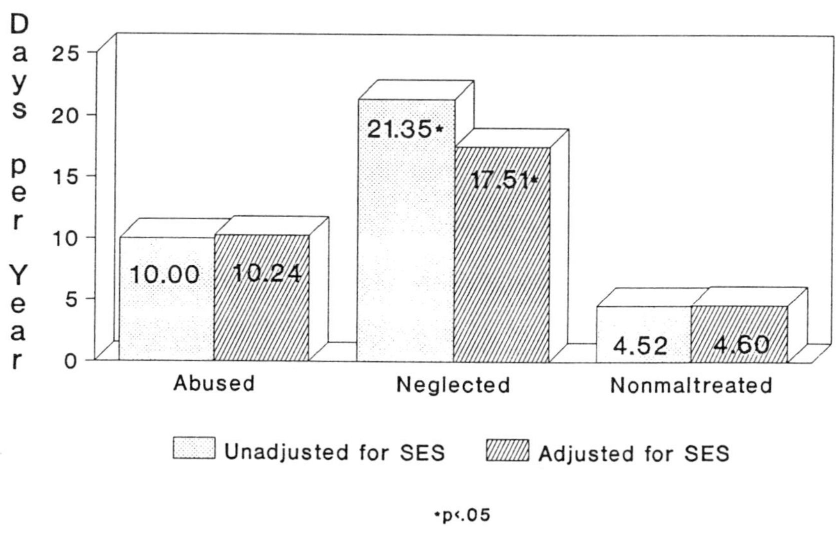

FIGURE 5. School Performance: Teacher Assessment of Performance

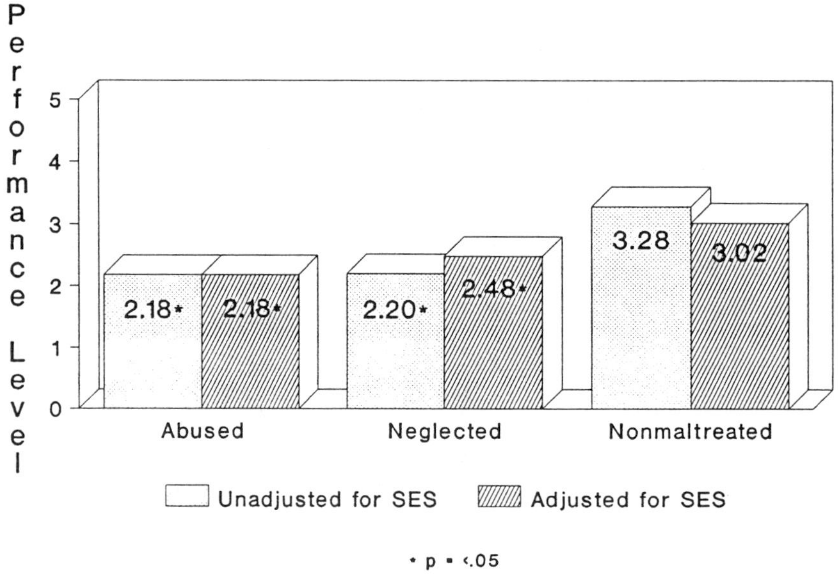

NOTE: Figures reflect combined scores of how well students were "working" and "learning" in the classroom.

FIGURE 6. Socioemotional Development: Problem Behavior at School (Teacher Assessment)

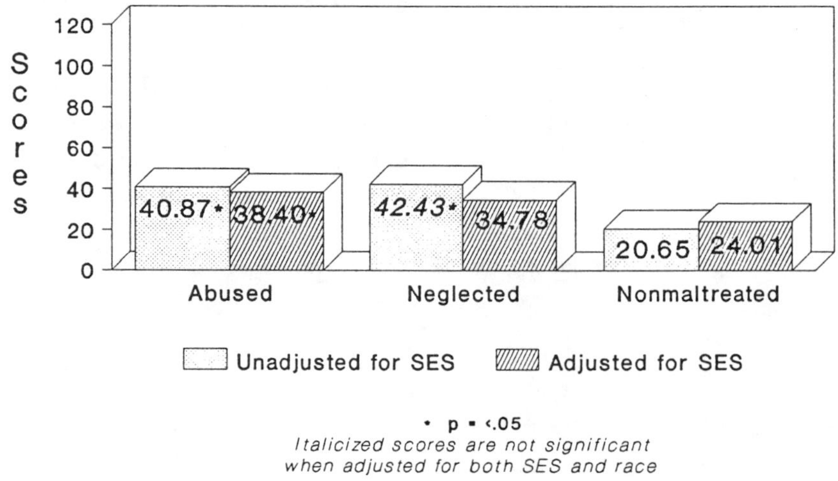

FIGURE 7. Socioemotional Development: Problem Behavior at Home (Parent Assessment)

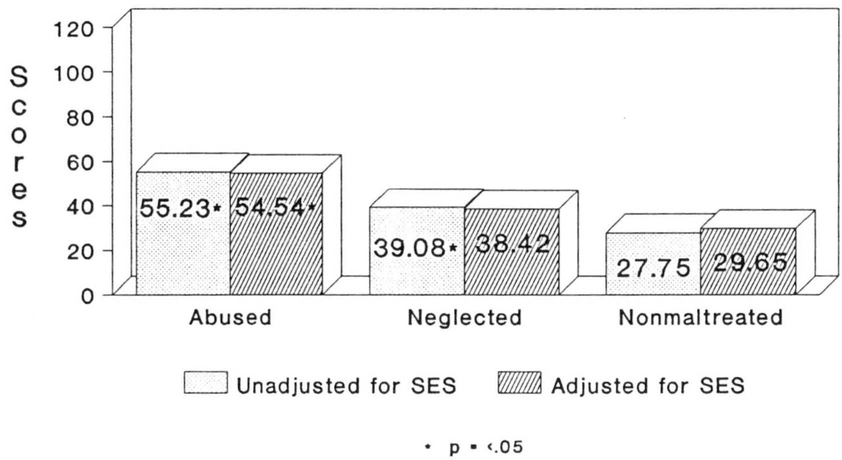

FIGURE 8. Socioemotional Development: Self-Concept

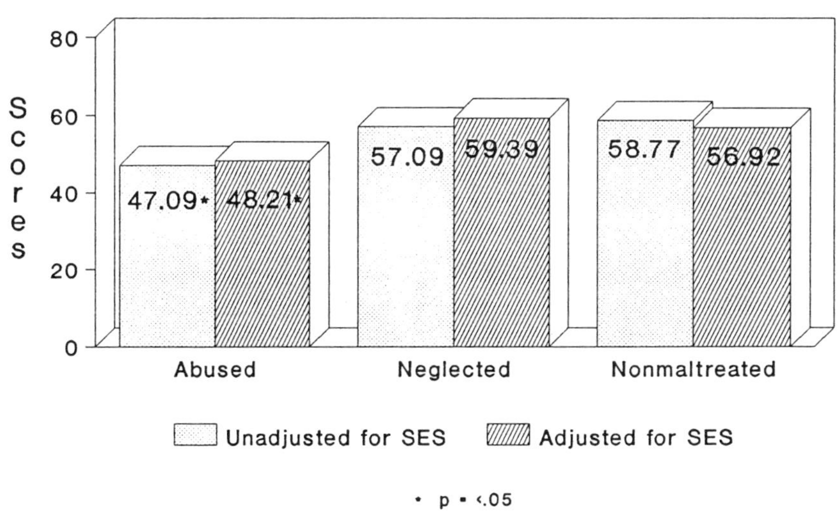

FIGURE 9. Socioemotional Development: Aggression

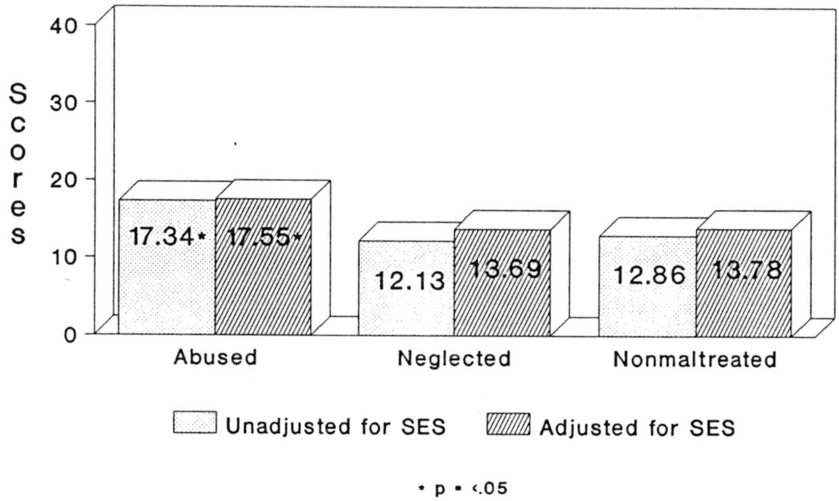

FIGURE 10. Socioemotional Development: School Maladjustment

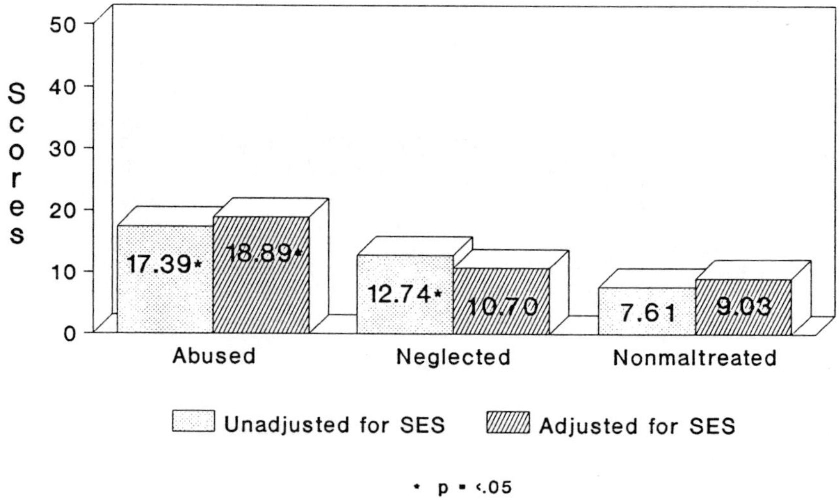

FIGURE 11. Socioemotional Development: Home Maladjustment

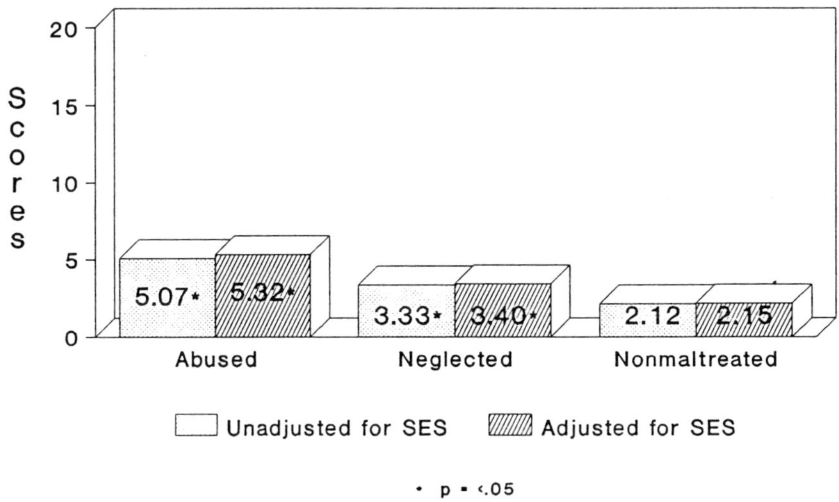

FIGURE 12. Socioemotional Development: Emotional Maladjustment

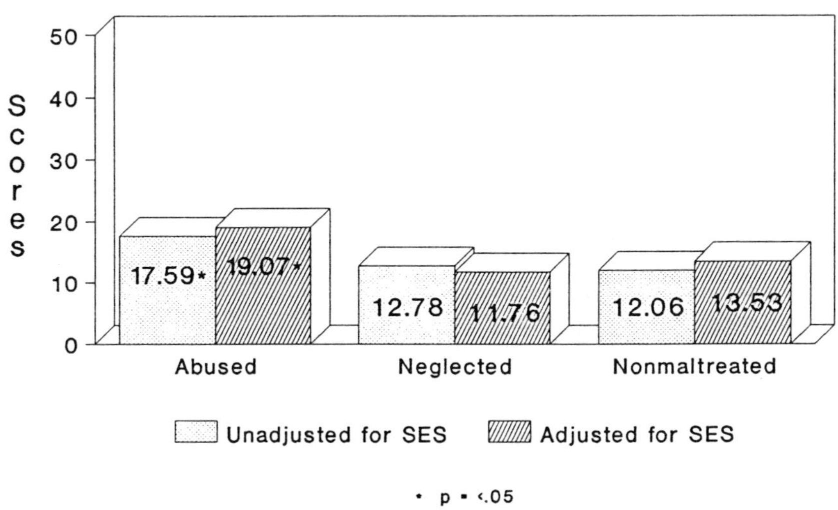

FIGURE 13. Socioemotional Development: Peer Maladjustment

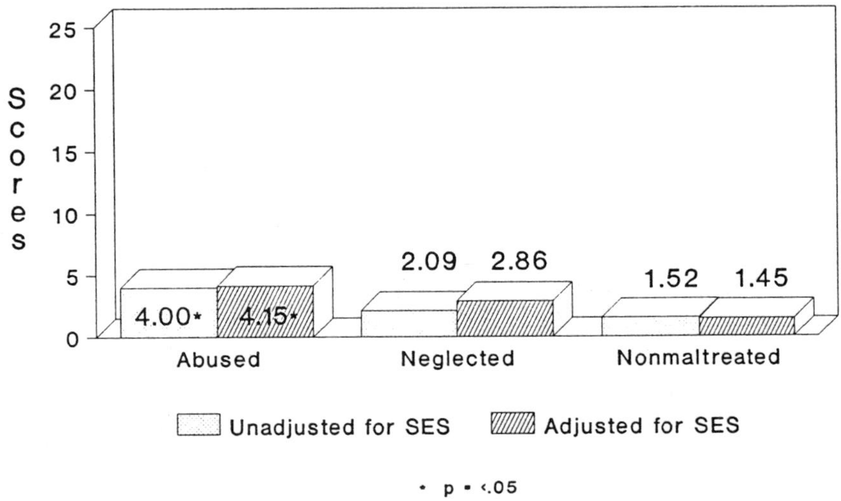

FIGURE 14. Socioemotional Development: Delinquency

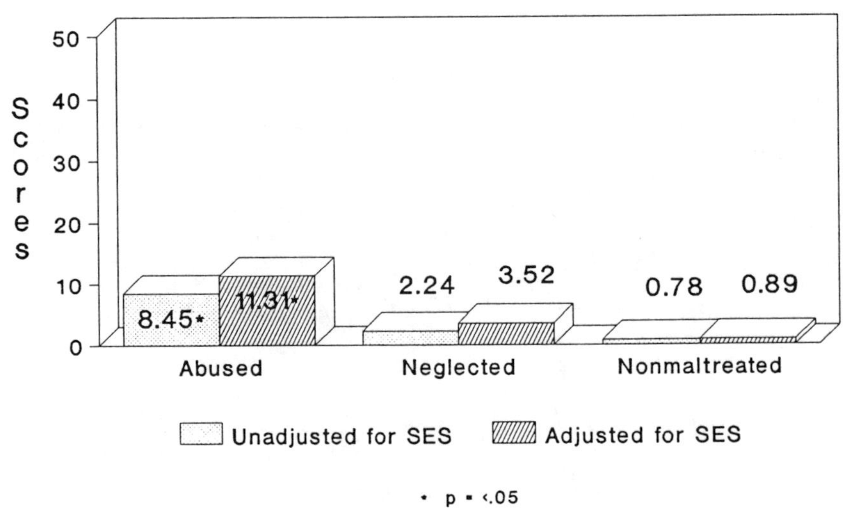

study ended, at least five abused children (23%) had dropped out of school, three (13%) had been placed in juvenile facilities for delinquents, three (13%) had become teenage mothers, one (5%) was pregnant, and another (5%) had been placed in a psychiatric facility after a suicide attempt. Chapter Four presents detailed findings about the physically abused children.

EFFECTS OF NEGLECT

Although the neglected children showed even more extreme academic delays than the abused children, they suffered no apparent socioemotional difficulties (see Figures 1-14; Tables B and C, Appendix). Parents, teachers, and the children themselves agreed that, aside from their school performance, these children were doing well. On nearly every measure of social relations and emotional adjustment, the neglected children were comparable to their nonmaltreated peers. On five of our nine socioemotional measures (self-concept, aggression, emotional adjustment, peer relationships, delinquency) the neglected children's scores were almost identical to those of their nonmaltreated schoolmates. The general absence of social and emotional problems for these children was completely unexpected, particularly because there is strong evidence that younger neglected children display a host of such problems.

Despite the apparent socioemotional strengths of our school-age neglected sample, academic difficulties were pronounced for these children. Their depressed test scores, teacher assessments of poor classroom performance, and high rates of absence set them strikingly apart from their nonmaltreated peers. Although the group showed significant improvement on school performance measures between initial and follow-up interviews (see Table D, Appendix), they were still performing far below their nonmaltreated peers. At least 10 (21%) had dropped out of school by the end of the study. Chapter Five gives a full account of our findings on neglected children.

ADAPTIVE STRENGTHS

Our findings suggest that both abused and neglected school-age children possess practical life skills appropriate to their age (see

Figures 15-17). We found remarkable similarities among the groups along all dimensions of adaptive functioning: motor skills, personal care skills (eating, toileting, dressing, self-care, and domestic skills), and community skills (time and punctuality, money and value, work skills, and home-community orientation). The implications of these results are extensive. Foremost, the finding suggests that maltreated children could benefit from therapeutic and educational strategies which emphasize a practical learn-by-doing approach.

EXPLANATION OF FIGURES

Figures 1-17 depict group differences on various measures of child development at the time of the first interviews. Each graph presents both raw scores and scores adjusted for SES (socioeconomic status), thus allowing for broad comparison of the abused and neglected children with normal peers. In most cases, the differ-

FIGURE 15. Adaptive Functioning: Motor Skills

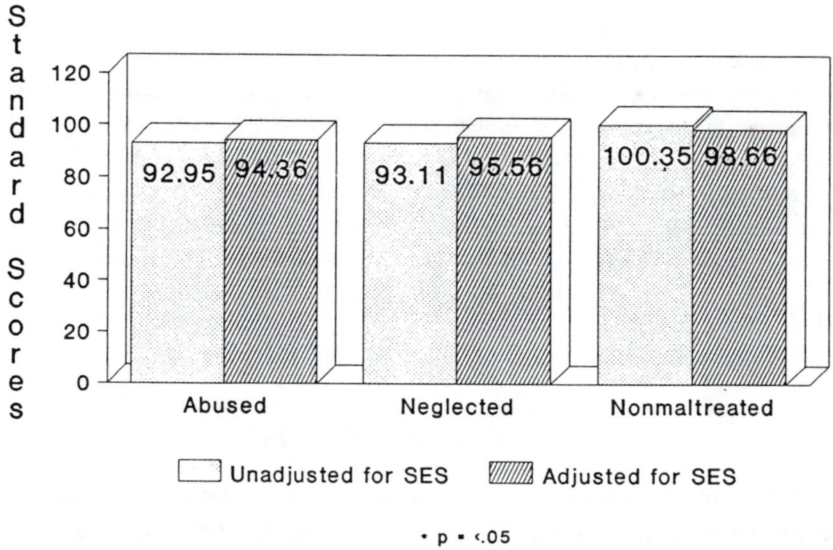

FIGURE 16. Adaptive Functioning: Personal Care Skills

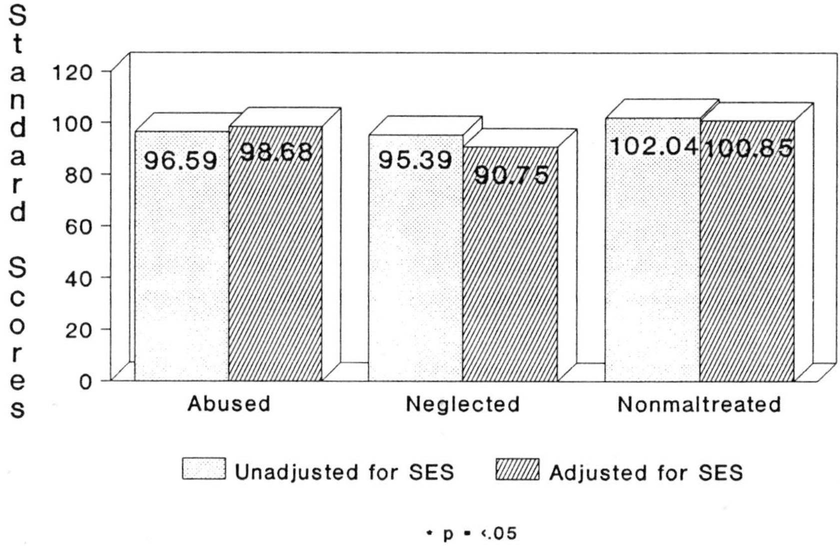

FIGURE 17. Adaptive Functioning: Community Skills

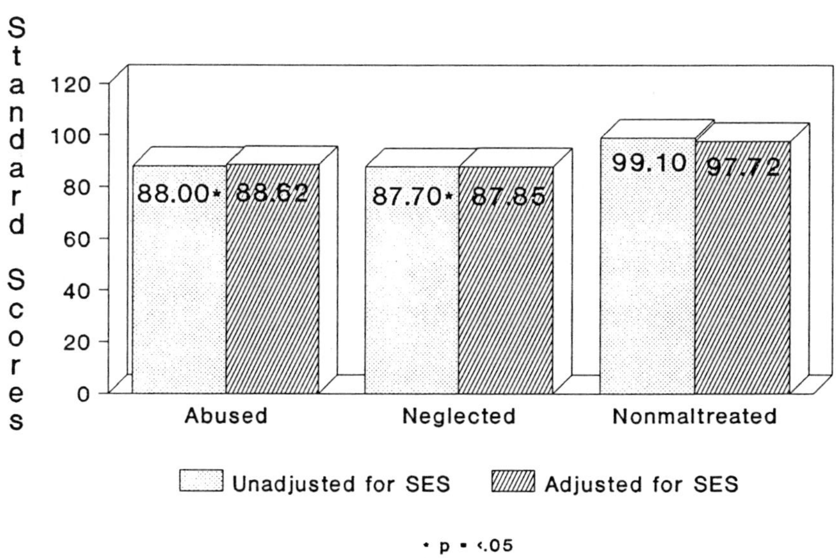

ences among the groups appear greater before adjustment for SES. This is because most of the maltreated children were from low SES families whereas the comparison group included children from all SES levels. Asterisks indicate statistically significant differences among the groups.

FAMILY FACTORS

Our findings regarding family factors were also provocative. Both abusive and neglectful families had experienced extreme stress from life events during the year prior to the first interviews. These high levels of stress were particularly related to the use of alcohol or drugs within the family, and, for neglectful families, to marital and interpersonal conflict. Further, children from the most stressed families functioned most poorly at school, at home, and with peers. The results suggest that family stress could have almost as much negative impact as physical abuse and, indeed, more negative impact than neglect on school-age children's socioemotional development.

Surprisingly, our hypothesis that maltreating families (especially neglectful families) were socially isolated was not supported by the data. All groups reported similar levels of social support from relatives, friends, neighbors, churches, and agencies. Parental depression was evident for abusive but not neglectful families. We found it intriguing that the children of depressed parents exhibited serious behavior problems both at home and school but did not display problems along any other dimension of socioemotional or academic development. Table E of the Appendix shows differences among the groups on family variables, and Table 3 shows significant predictors of poor functioning on various measures. Chapter Six explores our findings about family and background variables in depth.

MALTREATMENT HISTORIES

We were especially surprised at the general lack of differences among maltreated children as a result of their specific maltreatment

TABLE 3. Significant Predictors of Children's Poor Functioning of Abused or Neglected Children on Various Measures

Measure	Significant Predictors*
Poor overall school performance	Stressful life events
Problem behavior at school	Stressful life events Parental depression
Problem behavior at home	Parental depression More recent maltreatment
Low self-concept	More times in foster care
Elevated aggression	More times in foster care
Home maladjustment	Stressful life events More times in foster care
Emotional maladjustment	More times in foster care
Peer maladjustment	Stressful life events
Delinquency	Stressful life events Sexual abuse Number of forms of maltreatment

*significant predictors ($p < .05$) of outcome measures with SES controlled.

Note. Problem behavior = Child Behavior Checklist; self-concept = Piers-Harris Children's Self-Concept Scale; aggression = Jesness Manifest Aggression Subscale.

histories. Children whose maltreatment was more severe, chronic, or multiform were not faring more poorly on major dimensions of development. There was little apparent effect from sexual abuse or the length of time a child had spent in foster care. However, increases in the number of times a child had been placed in foster care were related to low self-concept, aggression, poor home adjustment, and poor emotional adjustment (see Table 3). It would appear that the effects of maltreatment are exacerbated by multiple placements.

SES AND RACE

Our research design enabled us to look at the effects of class on our sample. The results indicate that low SES is uniquely related to children's delays in community skills and to a lack of social support for the families we studied. Lower class children also experienced difficulties with poor school performance, problem behaviors in school and at home, low self-concept, aggression, poor adjustment in school and at home, poor emotional adjustment, delinquency, and family stress. However, there were no class differences with respect to the children's peer relations or their parents' marital relations. Further, there were no differences based on race except for teacher-reported problem behaviors (maltreated white students displayed far more school behavior problems than maltreated black students) and levels of social support (white families reported significantly less social support from kinship and community networks than black families).

SUMMARY

This chapter has presented key findings from The University of Georgia Child Maltreatment Project. School-age children who were physically abused displayed pervasive and severe academic and socioemotional problems. The neglected children differed little from comparison children on measures of socioemotional development, but displayed severe academic delays. Both groups of maltreated children showed unexpected strengths on measures of adaptive functioning. The figures included in this chapter show the initial differences among abused, neglected, and comparison children on major outcome variables.

High levels of stress, particularly stress related to alcohol or drug use by family members, characterized both abusive and neglectful families. Indeed, stress from life events predicted poor child functioning better than any other variable we examined except physical abuse. For abusive families, child behavior problems were specifically related to high levels of parental depression. There were surprisingly few effects from social isolation, severity or chronicity of maltreatment, or multiple forms of maltreatment, but multiple foster care placements were associated with child maladjustment. The results and their implications will be discussed in depth in the following chapters.

Chapter Four

Profile of the Physically Abused School-Age Child

We expected that the physically abused children we studied would be developmentally delayed compared to their nonmaltreated peers, but we hardly expected the extreme differences we found. These children displayed an overwhelming set of problems in school, at home, with peers, and in the community. With the notable exception of adaptive functioning, they were faring poorly on every major dimension of development we assessed, including school performance, adjustment, and behavior; home adjustment and behavior; self-concept; aggression; emotional adjustment; peer relationships; and delinquency. At follow-up, the abused children showed modest improvement on most measures, but their academic and behavioral problems at school had intensified.

Within a year of the initial interviews, many of the older children in the abuse group experienced severe life dysfunction: three (13%) had dropped out of school, two (9%) had been institutionalized in juvenile justice facilities, two (9%) had become teenage mothers, and one (5%) had been institutionalized in a psychiatric facility. None of the comparison group children had experienced such life disruptions. By the time the study ended, at least five (23%) abused children had dropped out of school, three (13%) had been in juvenile justice facilities, three (13%) had given birth, and one (5%) had become pregnant.

CASE PROFILE #1– ROSA: "I WISH I WERE DIFFERENT"

At the time our study began, 16-year-old Rosa lived with her natural parents and two younger brothers in a well-cared-for home. Both parents were employed full-time in blue collar jobs and attended church regularly. To our interviewer, Rosa looked like a typical teenager and seemed friendly and likeable. However, she had recently come to the attention of CPS authorities who found that she had been physically abused by her father. According to Rosa's mother, the family had experienced a high level of stress over the previous year. Apparently, the father began drinking heavily, marital conflict increased, Rosa ran away twice, and the parents divorced and remarried during this time. Rosa's mother showed signs of depression and a weak social network.

Information collected at the first set of interviews showed Rosa was faring poorly academically and socioemotionally. She was performing far below her ninth-grade classmates in English, reading, and math. She also tested lower than 90% of her peers on basic math skills and lower than 80% on basic language skills. She had been absent from school for 35 days during the previous year. Teachers, her mother, and Rosa herself agreed that she was markedly unhappy at school. Indeed, Rosa could not think of a single thing she liked about school.

Teachers identified a host of behavioral problems (among the highest scores received by any child in our study) and described her as depressed, underachieving, restless, inattentive, argumentative, confused, self-conscious, apathetic, impulsive, and feeling "worthless or inferior." Rosa's mother reported similar, though fewer, problems at home. Rosa rated herself as low in self-concept (e.g., "I wish I were different," "My looks bother me," and high in aggressive feelings (e.g., "Sometimes I feel like I want to beat up somebody"). She had appeared before juvenile court twice for delinquent offenses.

There was also evidence of emotional and adjustment problems. Rosa reported feeling sad nearly every day about family problems. She could not think of anything she liked about either parent, and she reported that she did not feel close to anyone in her family. She particularly singled out her father, saying she got along poorly with him because he was abusive. Although her mother claimed that Rosa had never used drugs or alcohol, Rosa reported using pot about once a week, and teachers noted that they were aware of the problem.

A few areas of strength emerged from the data. Rosa's peer relationships appeared to be successful: she had many friends, got along well with her peers, and saw herself as popular. In addition, although she lagged slightly behind her peers on community skills, she was above par in her motor and personal care skills.

A year after the initial interviews, CPS reported that Rosa's case was still open, though no new reports of maltreatment had occurred. However, Rosa had dropped out of school, and the family's telephone had been disconnected. Repeated attempts to locate Rosa and her family proved fruitless, and follow-up interviews were not conducted. At our final update, we received information that Rosa, now 19, had married and given birth to a child.

Rosa fits our profile of the physically abused school-age child in almost every respect: school failure, problem behaviors, low self-concept, high feelings of aggression, poor adjustment in school and at home, and delinquency are all part of the picture, as are the unexpected strengths in practical skills. Rosa differed only in her apparently successful peer adjustment. The high levels of stress (including serious alcohol problems) and parental depression in Rosa's family are also characteristic of the abusive families we studied.

POOR FUNCTIONING AT SCHOOL

At school, the abused children were functioning much more poorly than their nonmaltreated peers. By follow-up, their academic problems had become even more pronounced. Figures 1-5 and Table B show initial group differences on school measures, and Table D shows changes in overall school performance over time (figures cited are located in the previous chapter; tables cited are located in the Appendix).

The abused children scored significantly worse than comparison children on the math portion of the IOWA Test of Basic Skills (see Figure 2). Language scores were not substandard initially (see Figure 1), but fell precipitously by follow-up. Differences were significant when initial and follow-up information were analyzed together. According to teachers, the abused children were working and learning at significantly lower levels in the classroom than nonmaltreated children. They were also more likely to have repeated one or more grades, though their rates of absence were not significantly higher (see Figures 3-5). Older (age 12-16) abused boys showed the most severe academic delays whereas older abused girls were more likely to have dropped out of school between initial and follow-up interviews. Teachers reported that parents of abused youngsters showed little or no interest in their children's schooling (much less than parents of nonmaltreated children, and even less than neglecting parents).

Teachers reported a much higher number of behavior problems for abused children than for comparison children (see Figure 6; Table C), and these problems became more severe by follow-up (see Table D). The abused group's scores on the Child Behavior Checklist Teacher Form exceeded the "clinical range" cutoff point established for this instrument (i.e., the children scored similarly to children referred to mental health or special school services for behavioral and socioemotional problems). The problems identified by teachers covered a wide range of behaviors, including "externalizing" (e.g., aggressiveness, acting out) and "internalizing" (e.g., withdrawal, inattentiveness). The abused girls in the group were seen as particularly aggressive, delinquent, inattentive, nervous-overactive, and unpopular.

The abused children were also poorly adjusted at school, though they did show modest improvement in school adjustment between initial and follow-up interviews (see Figure 10; Tables C and D). Teachers and parents as well as the children themselves agreed that the abused children were unhappy in school, had trouble following school rules, and were unlikely to go as far in school as their nonmaltreated peers (27% of abused children were reportedly headed for college or technical school compared with 76% of nonmaltreated children). Older (age 12-16) abused boys were especially likely to show evidence of poor adjustment to school. Surprisingly, the abused children were no more likely than nonmaltreated children to have been paddled in school, suspended, or expelled.

This suggests that school personnel are, to a certain extent, sensitive to the special needs of abused children.

POOR FUNCTIONING AT HOME

In addition to their academic and socioemotional difficulties at school, the abused children displayed significant problem behaviors and maladjustment at home (see Figures 7 and 11; Table C). Parents reported a high number of problem behaviors for the abused youngsters, whose scores on the Child Behavior Checklist Parent Form (as well as the Teacher Form) placed them in the "clinical range" for this measure. Younger (age 8-11) abused boys were seen as particularly depressed, uncommunicative, obsessive-compulsive, withdrawn, hyperactive, aggressive, and delinquent. Older (age 12-16) abused girls were characterized as especially aggressive, delinquent, and cruel. At follow-up, parent-reported problems had decreased significantly, but the children were still perceived as far more problematic in the home than their nonmaltreated peers (see Table D).

Compared with nonmaltreated children, abused children were much more likely to report being unhappy with their families (38% of abused vs. 4% of nonmaltreated), and to report having problems getting along with their mothers (59% vs. 24%) and fathers (46% vs. 22%). Fourteen percent of abused children reported that they were not close to anyone in their family (vs. 1%), and 45% reported they were "picked on at home" (vs. 21%). The abused children were significantly more likely to report that they thought about running away from home (45% vs. 31%). When asked, "Do you wish there was anything different about your family?" abused children were significantly more likely than comparison children to wish either family members' behaviors would change (68% vs. 19%) or to change themselves (23% vs. 4%). They were somewhat more likely to want to change their families' composition (32% vs. 19%), but they were no more likely to wish for more material goods (23% vs. 22%). At follow-up, the abused children's home adjustment had improved somewhat (see Table D).

CASE PROFILE #2– ROBBIE: A POOR PROGNOSIS

According to CPS, 10-year-old Robbie had been physically abused by his mother's live-in boyfriend a number of times over a three-year period. The family had not officially been charged with neglect, but there was evidence that Robbie's physical and health needs were not being adequately met.

Instability and an extremely high level of stress characterized the family. When Robbie was interviewed, he reported that he lived with his mother, her boyfriend, and two younger brothers. The following month, however, his mother reported that her boyfriend no longer lived in the home, but five other extended family members did (including two adults, two teenagers, and a young child).

Trouble between Robbie's mother and her boyfriend had apparently involved an affair, heavy drinking, and arguments. Other recent stressors included job changes and difficulties with superiors at work (Robbie's mother worked in a factory), "getting into debt beyond means of repayment," and a period of homelessness. The family's support network seemed adequate, but Robbie's mother showed evidence of deep depression.

The family moved frequently (indeed, they moved from the area the following year and could not be located for inclusion at follow-up), and standardized test scores for Robbie were not on file. His teacher reported that Robbie was performing at grade level in most subjects, though he was working and learning at a slower rate than most of his second-grade classmates. According to both Robbie and his mother, he liked school very much and earned good grades, but was frequently in trouble with the teacher. His teacher confirmed that Robbie displayed a very high number of problem behaviors at school, including disobedience, irresponsibility, explosive behavior, irritability, sulking, and arguing. On the teacher form, she noted that he once "ran away from school, across traffic." Robbie reported that he was sent to the principal frequently, and that he had been paddled three times in the previous two school years.

At home, Robbie's behavior problems were more severe than those of any other child in the study. His mother identified extreme problems on all nine Child Behavior Checklist subscales for 6- to 11-year-old boys, especially the Aggressive, Uncommunicative, Social Withdrawal, and Hyperactive subscales. On the Aggressive scale, all 23 items were identified as problematic, with over half marked as serious problems, including the following: cruel to others, loud, brags, argues, shows off, and lies. She also reported that Robbie got along poorly with friends and family members. The primary form of punishment she used was "whippings" (almost all other parent respondents reported taking away privileges or, less often, scolding to be their usual disciplinary mode). On our adaptive scales, Robbie's mother rated him as lagging behind in motor skills (e.g., he could not catch a tennis ball with two hands or thread a needle) but functioning normally on personal care and community/work skills.

Although Robbie reported that he got along poorly with his mother, he said he was happy with his family and, indeed, could think of nothing he would change about his family. Further, he said he never thought about running away or hurting himself, and he reported few fears or worries. However, our interviewer noted that he was fidgety and restless throughout the interview and "reluctant to answer" many verbal questions. He was probably more forthright on written inventories: he scored low on self-concept (e.g., "I am different from other people," "I am [not] popular with boys") and high on feelings of aggression (e.g., "I have a real mean streak in me").

Gaps in our data on Robbie's school performance limit our ability to assess his academic development. Although his current school performance seemed satisfactory, we obtained no standardized scores to anchor our more subjective data. If Robbie fits the profile we found for physically abused children, these scores would be quite low. He certainly fits the profile in other respects: he was severely impaired socioemotionally (but could function normally on most practical life skills), and his family was characterized by high stress and parental depression.

At last report, Robbie and his family had returned to the community. The family situation remained chaotic. After a brief placement in foster care, a judge returned Robbie to his mother's custody against CPS recommendations. Without intensive concrete and therapeutic services, the prognosis for Robbie and his family must be considered poor.

POOR SELF-CONCEPT AND EMOTIONAL MALADJUSTMENT

The abused children scored much lower on self-concept and emotional adjustment than nonmaltreated children (see Figures 8 and 12; Table C). Compared with national norms established for the Piers-Harris Children's Self-Concept Scale, the abused group's raw score placed them in the 33rd percentile of all children, while the comparison group scored in the 65th percentile. Abused children scored lower on all six subscales of the Piers-Harris: Behavior, Intellectual, Physical, Anxiety, Popularity, and Happiness and Satisfaction. Their scores were especially low on the Behavior subscale (e.g., "I do many bad things," "I get into a lot of fights," "I am often mean to other people") and on the Happiness and Satisfaction subscale (e.g., "I am unhappy," "I wish I were different," "I am [not] lucky").

The abused children were much more likely than nonmaltreated children to have thought about killing themselves (31% vs. 9%), or to have actually attempted suicide (27% vs. 1%). They reported pervasive feelings of sadness (feeling sad nearly every day; 41% vs. 9%), significantly more sleep difficulties (59% vs. 40%) and appetite problems (particularly overeating; 23% vs. 9%), and slightly more problems with frequent stomachaches or headaches (32% vs. 25%) and nightmares (9% vs. 4%). Abused children were somewhat more likely than comparison children to report feeling nervous a lot (64% vs. 43%) and that terrible things would happen to them (68% vs. 53%). A significant number reported losing their tempers nearly every day (27% vs. 6%).

On the other hand, abused children reported fewer fears and worries than nonmaltreated children. They were less likely to fear animals (15% vs. 44%), heights (20% vs. 37%), strangers (60% vs.

84%), being in closed spaces (20% vs. 26%), or being away from home (20% vs. 26%), but they were significantly more likely to fear their parents (20% vs. 8%). They worried less about bad storms or fires (33% vs. 39%), being lost or kidnapped (52% vs. 63%), or parents fighting (48% vs. 53%), divorcing (33% vs. 48%), or dying (71% vs. 85%), but they worried slightly more about parents becoming sick (62% vs. 56%). At follow-up, the abused children showed modest improvement of both self-concept and emotional adjustment (see Figure D).

POOR PEER RELATIONSHIPS

Compared with nonmaltreated children, the abused children's peer relationships were troubled, though they improved somewhat by follow-up (see Figure 13; Tables C and D). Parents reported that 32% of the abused children got along "poorly" or "very poorly" with other children (vs. 0% of nonmaltreated children). Nearly half of the abused children described themselves as unpopular (vs. 37%), and 41% found it hard to make friends (vs. 20%). Some 20% of the abuse group (vs. 3%) could not think of any activities they engaged in with their friends other than "hanging out." For 14% of the abused children (vs. 3%), their best friends were two or more years older. However, the abused children had as many friends as nonmaltreated children and reportedly spent more time with friends. Thus, despite their peer relationship difficulties, we might speculate that the abused children were attempting to transfer their need for acceptance from their families to friendship networks.

AGGRESSION AND DELINQUENCY

The abused group's excessive aggression and delinquency were substantiated by various measures and sources. Parents and teachers identified a range of aggressive and delinquent behaviors for the abused children, especially abused girls. The children themselves reported a much higher level of aggressive feelings than nonmaltreated children (see Figure 9; Table C) on the Jesness Manifest

Aggression Subscale (e.g., "A person like me fights first and asks questions later," "Sometimes it's fun to steal something," "I can't seem to take much kidding or teasing").

Abused children had also engaged in considerably more delinquent activities than comparison children (see Figure 14; Table C). They were much more likely to have appeared in juvenile court than nonmaltreated children (47% vs. 3%), and they admitted to far more offenses, including:

- skipping school (29% vs. 0%)
- stealing (45% vs. 13%)
- reckless driving (14% vs. 0%)
- threatening others to get money (14% vs. 1%)
- purse-snatching (5% vs. 0%)
- robbery (9% vs. 0%)
- physically hitting others (41% vs. 16%)
- vandalizing property (18% vs. 3%)
- breaking into a house, car, or building (14% vs. 0%)
- fire-setting (9% vs. 1%).

The abused children were also much more likely to have used drugs or alcohol (41% vs. 9%), and 13% (vs. 0%) admitted to using drugs or alcohol once a week or more.

Although the children showed slight improvement on our aggression and delinquency measures by follow-up (see Table D), the severity of their problems in these areas is cause for particular concern because of the poor prognosis for children with antisocial disorders. When aggressive and delinquent behaviors appear during childhood, they are likely to extend into adulthood in the form of criminal behavior, alcoholism, drug addiction, and psychosis.[1]

CASE PROFILE #3–
ERIC: ABUSED AND NEGLECTED

Eric, 14, had been both physically abused and neglected within the previous 18 months. The abuse charge stemmed from a severe beating by his 18-year-old brother. Neglect charges were apparently based on a lack of utilities and parental supervision. At the time of our first set of interviews, Eric lived with his mother and three brothers in an unpretentious but well-cared-for home. His mother reported high levels of stress for the previous year, largely stemming from problems with unemployment, job changes, alcohol or drug use by family members, moving, and an increase in family arguments. Her social support network was barely adequate, and she showed evidence of depression.

Eric appeared sad during his interview, and he frequently gave brief answers or responded "I don't know." The information we collected showed that he was faring poorly at school, scoring far below average on standardized tests and earning mostly F's. He attributed his poor grades to a lack of effort rather than a lack of ability. He had been absent 16 days during the previous school year. He said he disliked school and could not say how far he would go in school, though his mother expected him to graduate. Eric's teachers reported a high number of problem behaviors in the classroom, including comments such as "acts too young for his age," "can't concentrate," and "hangs with others who get in trouble." The same problems were also reported by Eric's mother, along with descriptions of "stubborn," "secretive," and "likes to be alone."

Eric's self-concept was quite low (e.g., "I feel left out of things," "I am [not] good-looking," "I forget what I learn"), and he reported higher-than-normal feelings of aggression (e.g., "Sometimes it's fun to steal something"). He had appeared before juvenile court for a delinquency offense, and he admitted to stealing, skipping school, vandalizing property, breaking and entering, and setting a fire. He also reported that he had run away and that he used drugs or alcohol, though infrequently. On adaptive measures, he was performing below par, especially on community skills involving money and finding his way around town. However, he appeared to have an adequate friendship network.

Between initial and follow-up interviews, new charges of maltreatment were substantiated, and Eric was placed in a boys' home in a different county. Our follow-up interviews were conducted with Eric at his new school and with a house parent at the boys' home. Most follow-up measures showed evidence of deterioration from the previous year, especially in the areas of school performance and adjustment, and delinquency (he had appeared again in juvenile court and now reported drinking or using drugs on a weekly basis). His peer relationships were apparently disrupted by the move and were no longer satisfactory.

Unfortunately, Eric's new school was unable to provide completed teacher reports, so we can only speculate as to his school behavior at follow-up. However, his house parent reported that Eric was in trouble at school frequently ("every two or three days"), and that he displayed a very high number of problem behaviors in the home. These included all the problems noted above from the previous year and a rash of new problems involving aggressive and nervous behaviors. We received no information about Eric at our final update, but it seems unlikely that his problems have been resolved.

Eric's case illustrates our finding that school-age children who have been both abused and neglected fit with our abuse group rather than with our neglect group. While all the maltreated children showed similar academic delays, only the abused children were socioemotionally impaired. Eric differed from both groups in that he displayed poor adaptive functioning (most of the maltreated children we studied were functioning normally on adaptive measures).

STRONG IN PRACTICAL SKILLS

Surprisingly, the abused children we studied were functioning as well as nonmaltreated children on a variety of practical skills, including gross and fine motor skills (see Figure 15), personal care skills (eating, toileting, dressing, self-care, and domestic skills; see Figure 16), and community skills (time and punctuality, money and value, work skills, and home-community orientation; see Figure 17). At follow-up, their personal care and community skills had declined somewhat (not significantly), but their motor skills had improved (see Table D).

Although the validity of these results may be suspect because we relied on parent reports of the children's adaptive behaviors rather than direct testing or observation, we believe the results are credible. It makes intuitive sense that abused children would learn to adapt in functional ways to their environments. Abusive parents may demand children's compliance in areas of self-care, chores, and community expectations. Since the implications of our finding are extensive, future research efforts should assess abused children's adaptive functioning through direct testing, observation, and collateral sources.

IMPLICATIONS

Our findings indicate that the consequences of physical abuse are severe for school-age children. The academic and socioemotional problems displayed by the abused children in our study will certainly not disappear without the implementation of a range of child-centered intervention services. With the exception of school performance and school behavior, the abused children did show improvement on our measures over the course of the study. However, they were still functioning much more poorly than their non-maltreated peers at follow-up in every domain of academic and socioemotional functioning. Considering the magnitude of difficulties, it seems likely that many of the younger abused children who participated in the study will, without intensive treatment services, follow their adolescent counterparts by experiencing major life disturbances, especially school failure or dropping out.

It is notable that improvements between initial and follow-up interviews were not apparent at school. It may be that changes occur more slowly in the school setting or that a child's reputation as a slow learner or behavior problem sets up self-fulfilling negative expectations among teachers. Casework services may need to include greater collaboration with schools, perhaps through a school social worker, in order for improved functioning to become evident in the classroom.

The abused children we studied are in need of remedial and

therapeutic services to overcome the pervasive and enduring effects of abuse. Specific deficits in math, language, and other academic subjects should be addressed through such means as tutoring, self-paced lessons, a system of clear and consistent performance standards, and immediate rewards for incremental achievements. Teacher aides and summer remediation programs (tuition-free for those unable to pay) could also boost performance. A recent report sponsored by the Carnegie Corporation, entitled *Turning Points: Preparing American Youth for the 21st Century,* calls for sweeping educational reforms to address the kinds of school problems displayed by both the abused and the neglected children in our study.[2] The Carnegie report's recommendations include restructuring large schools into smaller units, eliminating tracking, promoting cooperative learning through team teaching, and assigning an advisor to each student.

Many abused children may be eligible for special education services because of their academic or socioemotional difficulties, and this possibility should be assessed when abuse has been identified. However, adolescents and preadolescents often have a strong resistance to special class placement. The older abused child may need a flexible program that allows for a considerable degree of mainstreaming. Vocational education may be a key element of such a program. Our finding of unexpected strength in the functional behaviors of maltreated children suggests that a learn-by-doing approach and a concentration on practical skills should be adopted for these children.

Special education services are more likely to be available for academically delayed than socioemotionally impaired (SEI) children. In principle, the Education for All Handicapped Children Act provides federal funds for schools to establish SEI classes in which specially trained teacher-counselors focus on academic, social, and prevocational-vocational skills.[3] The classes teach self-responsibility through such means as reality therapy, behavioral point systems, time-out, concrete and social reinforcers, and group counseling. Parents are involved through problem-solving sessions that promote collaboration and unified parent-child initiatives. Goals, expectations, roles, and time limits are spelled out in the Individualized Education Program (IEP) developed for each special education student. Through IEP directives, children may be mainstreamed with special conditions set, or they may attend special classes for several hours or all day. Thus far, few school districts have utilized special education funds for SEI classes, but the rising number of problem students over the past decade may stimulate efforts in this direction.

Given the severity of the abused children's socioemotional problems, mental health services seem essential for these children. Assessment procedures should focus particularly on problem behavior; aggression; delinquency; adjustment in school, at home, and with peers; and should include evaluation of suicidal tendencies and substance abuse.

Individual therapy for the abused child should focus on helping the victim to self-disclose about the trauma and to verbalize feelings.[4] Art, writing, and bibliotherapy are useful in encouraging such expression in the older child. However, insight-oriented therapy is costly and time consuming, and may not be sufficient to correct severe developmental deficits. Effective intervention is likely to require social, cognitive, and behavioral therapeutic approaches. Group counseling; family counseling; training in social skills, life skills, and problem-solving skills; peer counseling; recreational programs; temporary therapeutic respite care; and vocational counseling have all been used to address the kinds of socioemotional problems displayed by school-age abused children.[5]

Of course, any intervention must be implemented within the context of the child's larger environment. Given the transactional nature of family systems, parent and child services must be integrated. Practitioners must anticipate and ward off possible negative familial repercussions of the child's positive behavior change (e.g., verbal initiatives made by the child may be punished by parents who are not actively involved in the treatment process).

CASE PROFILES #4– BRIEF UPDATES ON PHYSICAL ABUSE CASES

The following information was provided by CPS and/or school system personnel approximately two years after our final interviews. The information is spotty, and we have no updated information at all on seven abused children (31%; three girls, four boys). (Note: The names given are fictitious.)

- Alex (now 11) is in the fifth grade and is displaying severe behavior problems. He comes to school "very dirty and unkempt." His stepfather is "emotionally abusive" to school staff, and school and CPS personnel suspect, but have not confirmed, new physical abuse by the stepfather.
- Tara (11) is performing poorly in the fourth grade and "resists doing her work more than in previous years." Teachers express concern that she "has very advanced sexual information for her age [which she] openly talks about in front of peers and teachers."
- Robbie (12; see Case Profile #2–Robbie: A Poor Prognosis) is in school (details unknown). His family situation remains chaotic; after a brief placement in foster care a judge returned custody to the mother against CPS recommendations.
- Sammie (12) has been placed in a behavior disorders class at fifth-grade level. There have been new reports of physical abuse by his father.
- Christopher (13) is in the sixth grade and "has not missed a day of school this school year." However, school personnel are aware of problems in the family and "may have to report to [CPS] soon."
- Mark (14) is doing "better than ever" in a boys' home out-of-county. His mother is in prison.
- Cheryl (15) is in the ninth grade. Her family has moved a number of times in the last few years, and there have been marital and financial troubles. Cheryl has reportedly become involved with a Satanic cult and has experimented with hallucinogenic drugs. She has "claimed to be pregnant" twice this school year and plans to marry in a few months.
- Barbara (16) was on the honor roll while in foster care, but she was returned home and is currently failing most of her classes. She is working, and she ran away with an older boy for several days.

- Pam (17) was in a juvenile facility for delinquents at the time of our follow-up interviews. She was subsequently returned to her mother's custody, gave birth to a child, and committed new juvenile offenses. She has been placed in another juvenile facility and her baby is currently in foster care.
- Elizabeth (17) has been in a residential treatment facility for drug abuse and in a juvenile detention facility for unruly behavior. School officials also report rebellious behavior (grade level unknown). She has had an abortion and a miscarriage and admits to cocaine use.
- Jimmy (17) is in a juvenile facility for delinquent boys.
- Janet (17) is in school (details unknown) and is "doing fine" since her parents divorced.
- Paula (18) was in a residential psychiatric facility at the time of our follow-up interviews. After returning to her family she dropped out of school. Her current whereabouts are unknown.
- Steven (19) was placed with an older sister and is in a self-contained special education class in 11th grade.
- Wanda (19) graduated from high school and is enrolled in a technical school. After her alcoholic mother died she was placed with an aunt, but she now lives on her own.
- Missy (19) dropped out of school, is married, and has a child.
- Rosa (19; see Case Profile #1–Rosa: "I Wish I Were Different") dropped out of school in ninth grade, is married, and has a child.

CONCLUSION

This chapter has detailed the severe academic and socioemotional problems of school-age children who have been physically abused. We discussed a range of remedial and therapeutic services these children need if they are to enter adulthood (and parenthood) with confidence, motivation, and the skills required for success. Later chapters will focus on systemic obstacles to needed treatment services and what we must do to ensure appropriate services for abused school-age children.

NOTES

1. L.N. Robins, "Sturdy Childhood Predictors of Adult Antisocial Behavior: Replications from Longitudinal Studies," *Psychological Medicine* 8 (1978): 611-22; C. S. Widom, "Child Abuse, Neglect, and Adult Behavior: Research Design and Findings on Criminality, Violence, and Child Abuse," *American Journal of Orthopsychiatry* 59 (1989): 355-67.

2. Carnegie Corporation, *Turning Points: Preparing American Youth for the 21st Century* (New York: Carnegie Corporation, 1989).

3. W.C. Morse, *The Education and Treatment of Socioemotionally Impaired Children and Youth* (Syracuse: Syracuse University Press, 1985).

4. C.M. Mouzakitis and R. Varghese, eds., *Social Work Treatment with Abused and Neglected Children* (Springfield, IL: Charles C Thomas, 1988); C.F. Schaefer and K.J. O'Connor, eds., *Handbook of Play Therapy* (New York: John Wiley, 1983).

5. D. Daro, *Confronting Child Abuse: Research for Effective Program Design* (New York: Free Press, 1988); C.E. Walker and B.L. Bonner, *The Physically and Sexually Abused Child: Evaluation and Treatment* (New York: Pergamon, 1988); G.R. Patterson, *A Social Learning Approach,* vol. 3, *Coercive Family Process* (Eugene, OR: Castalia, 1982); D.K. Jewell, *Confronting Child Abuse Through Recreation* (Springfield, IL: Charles C Thomas, 1989); S.D. Euster, V.P. Ward, J.G. Varner, and G.L. Euster, "Life Skills Group for Adolescent Foster Children," *Child Welfare* 63, no. 1 (1984): 27-36; P. Shelton, "Separation and Treatment of Child-Abusing Families," *Family Therapy* 9, no. 1 (1982): 53-59; P. Dale, T. Morrison, M. Davies, P. Noyes, and W. Roberts, "A Family-Therapy Approach to Child Abuse: Countering Resistance," *Journal of Family Therapy* 5 (1983): 117-43.

Chapter Five

Profile of the Neglected School-Age Child

We expected that the neglected children's scores would be similar to those of abused children on our various measures of child development, but this was true only on tests of academic and adaptive functioning. Both neglected and abused children were performing poorly at school but adequately in terms of practical skills. However, the two groups diverged sharply on socioemotional measures. The severe and pervasive socioemotional problems displayed by physically abused children were absent for neglected children, who appeared, overall, to be as happy and well adjusted as their nonmaltreated peers.

CASE PROFILE #5– EDDIE: NEGLECTED BUT HAPPY?

Ten-year-old Eddie and his two brothers lived with their never-married mother, an unskilled worker with an eighth-grade education. He (and presumably his brothers) was considered neglected by CPS on the basis of lack of supervision, inconsistent discipline, and inadequate household furnishings (the lack of a telephone meant we had to schedule the parent interview by mail). Although the caseworker reported that sanitation and physical safety in the home were "adequate," our interviewer found the apartment in which the family resided to be in a state of serious disrepair ("unsafe to live in"). Further, the interviewer reported "Roaches crawled on walls and mice [scurried] on the floor throughout this interview. A worker of fainter heart wouldn't have lasted the whole interview–I barely did!"

Two weeks before the home visit, the interviewer had met with Eddie at school and found him to be friendly, likeable ("very!"), well adjusted, and apparently happy with his family situation. Indeed, Eddie could think of nothing he would change about his family and nothing he didn't like about his mother. On most of our socioemotional and functional measures he appeared well adjusted and capable. However, like the overwhelming majority of our neglected sample, he was receiving F's in the third grade, was frequently absent, and had repeated one grade. His teacher identified a moderate number of problems on the Child Behavior Checklist. These revolved around academic difficulties and distractibility; however, Eddie was reportedly behaving appropriately and seemed happy in school. Despite his academic difficulties, Eddie said he liked school "a lot" and thought he would earn a college degree someday.

His mother thought high school was as far as he would go, but she presented Eddie as normal in every way–few problems, many friends, good practical skills, and good relationships with family and friends. She considered herself a happy person as well and had an active and dependable social network. However, she did report high levels of job-related stress for the previous year, including a period of unemployment and money problems before finding another job.

At follow-up, Eddie was repeating third grade, but he was making A's and B's this time and displaying few problem behaviors. He still liked school but had given up his college aspirations. On every socioemotional and functional measure he appeared normal, happy, and capable. The only hint of problems appeared on the self-concept scale. Eddie changed his answer on 10 items, in each case giving a more positive response than the erased original. His mother, still living at the same address (and still without a phone), gave a glowing report of Eddie's well-being and behavior. She, however, was unemployed again because of trouble with superiors. She was "unsure" whether she still considered herself a happy person, though her social network was even more extensive than the previous year. We have no information on Eddie's current school status, but his CPS case has been closed.

Eddie typifies the neglected children in our study. Despite severe school problems, he appeared to be functioning normally on most socioemotional and functional measures, and at follow-up his academic problems had diminished. Like most neglectful families in the study, Eddie's family was characterized by stress but not by depression or lack of social support. For neglected children like Eddie, intervention should focus on strengthening academic skills and alleviating family stress.

ACADEMIC PROBLEMS

Academic failure emerged as the single most dramatic and consistent risk factor for school-age neglected children, who scored far below their nonmaltreated peers on school performance measures. Figures 1-5 and Table B show group differences on school measures at initial data collection (figures cited are located in Chapter Three; tables cited are located in the Appendix).

The neglected children's raw scores on standardized tests of language, math, and reading skills were much lower even than those of abused children. On the Iowa Test of Basic Skills, the neglected children's scores placed them in the 29th percentile on language skills compared with the 44th percentile for abused children and the 67th for comparison children (see Figure 1). On math skills, their scores placed them in the 28th percentile compared with the 42nd percentile for abused children and the 73rd for comparison children (see Figure 2). Scores on the reading portion of the Georgia Criterion Reference Test were also significantly lower for neglected children (however, the lack of difference on the math portion of the Georgia CRT calls into question the ability of this test to discriminate among high and low achievers). Teacher reports confirmed that the neglected children were working and learning at lower levels than with other children in the classroom (see Figure 5). Older (age 12-16) black males in the neglect group were especially lagging in academic skills.

The neglect group's rate of absence was nearly five times that of the comparison group (21.35 days for the previous year vs. 4.5 days; see Figure 4), and educational aspirations for the group were quite low. Although three-fourths of comparison parents expected their children to pursue education beyond a high school diploma, only one fourth of neglect group parents expected their children to go to college or trade school. By follow-up, two (4%) of the neglected children had dropped out of school (vs. none of the comparison children), and at least ten (21%) neglected children had dropped out at last report.

Of the neglected children, 60% had repeated one or more grades compared with 24% of comparison children. Surprisingly, this sizable difference was not statistically significant when SES (socioeconomic status) differences between the groups were taken into account (see Figure 3). The lack of significance suggests that grade retention is more strongly associated with SES than with academic performance for the children we studied. Informal discussions with school administrators confirmed that low SES students who perform poorly academically but "are doing the best they can do" are frequently given social promotions. It is also possible that more of the neglected children had been placed in special education classes and were subsequently promoted at higher rates than their academic performance would have allowed in regular classes. By federal law, school systems are prohibited from releasing information about special education histories, thus this factor could not be included in the data analysis.

For the most part, the neglected children's school problems were confined to academic difficulties; the group as a whole did not display behavior or adjustment problems in the classroom. And, encouragingly, the neglected children showed significantly improved school performance between initial and follow-up interviews (see Table D). Their second-year scores on standardized tests of language, reading, and math skills were all higher than the previous year. On the Iowa Test, improvements in language skills moved them from the 29th to the 40th percentile, and improvements in math skills moved them from the 28th to the 37th percentile. By contrast, scores for both abused and comparison children dropped between initial and follow-up investigation. The neglected children, however, still scored far below comparison children on overall school performance at follow-up, and teachers reported that these children were working and learning at lower levels than the year before.

CASE PROFILE #6– TAMMY: MAKING PROGRESS

According to CPS, nine-year-old Tammy was a neglected child. Specific problems involved inadequacies of household sanitation, personal hygiene, clothing, household furnishings, and supervision. Tammy had recently moved to the area with her mother, father, and baby sister. They lived in a housing project described by our interviewer as a slum district. Neither parent had more than a grade-school education, the mother had never worked, and total family income was under $10,000 a year.

Tammy's father, a factory worker, completed both the initial and follow-up interviews. He reported that the family had experienced a high level of stress the year before the first interview, including unemployment, moving, and legal problems. There was evidence of marital conflict (but not parental depression), and social support for the family was minimal.

Academically, Tammy's performance was far below average. She scored in the lowest 12th percentile in basic language skills and in the lowest 16th percentile in basic math skills. However, she said she liked school and, unlike most of the neglected children we studied, was seldom absent. She had repeated first grade, was currently in second, and expected to complete only nine years of schooling, though her father expected that she would graduate.

Tammy saw herself as well adjusted, with many friends, a happy home life, a good self-concept, and few aggressive impulses. However, she reported sleep and nightmare problems and thought she worried more than most kids about such things as accidents; storms; being lost or kidnapped; and parents fighting, divorcing, or being harmed. Her father also expressed concern over her nightmares and worrying, but he reported few behavior problems at home. However, he informed the interviewer that Tammy was being treated with Ritalin for hyperactivity.

On the teacher form, Tammy's teacher noted that when Tammy took her medication, behavior problems at school were minimal, but that numerous problems surfaced when she did not. These included restlessness, nervousness, disobedience, stubbornness, inattentiveness, clowning, and unpredictability. Apparently this circumstance occurred infrequently, although our interviewer reported that Tammy was tense, fidgety, and restless during both interview sessions.

Unlike most of the maltreated children in this study, Tammy scored far below her peers on all three measures of adaptive behavior. Particular problems were noted in the areas of gross motor skills, eating and domestic skills, money and value, work skills, and community skills. For example, she could not ride a bicycle; open a can with a can opener; sweep the floor with a broom; state the day, month, and year of her birth; or count 50 objects without stopping.

At follow-up, Tammy's school performance had improved significantly, and she had gone from being a C to a B student. She was still a worrier but reported fewer sleep disturbances and nightmares now. She appeared happy and well adjusted, though she still lagged behind her peers on adaptive skills. The family's situation had also improved: only minor stressors were reported and marital conflicts seemed to have been resolved. However, the family was still socially isolated from the community.

Tammy's hyperactivity, sleep disturbance, worries, and lags in adaptive skills are not typical of our neglected sample, but in other ways she fits the profile of the school-age neglected child. Like most of the neglected children we studied, Tammy was struggling academically, but showed significant improvement at follow-up. She also displayed few socioemotional problems at school, at home, in the community, or with peers. And, like most of the neglectful families, Tammy's family had experienced high levels of stress and marital conflict (their persistent lack of social support was atypical, however). The improvements in Tammy and her family between the initial and follow-up interviews may reflect the provision of CPS services to the family.

NORMAL ADAPTIVE SKILLS

Like the abused children, the neglected children in our study were functioning as well as nonmaltreated children in such areas as gross and fine motor skills, personal care and domestic skills, and community/work skills (see Figures 15-17). At follow-up, their scores had improved on all domains, especially motor skills (see Table D). These findings suggest that older neglected children manage to learn a variety of practical skills needed for survival. Because our study was the first to examine the adaptive functioning of school-age maltreated children, this finding should not be accepted as gospel without further research. However, an important tentative implication of our study is that maltreated children may profit from a learn-by-doing approach at school and a concentration on practical skills as opposed to seatwork.

SOCIOEMOTIONAL STRENGTHS

Perhaps the most surprising and provocative finding of our study involves the striking contrast between abused and neglected school-age children on socioemotional measures (see Figures 6-14; Table C). Whereas abused children scored significantly worse than comparison children on all nine of our socioemotional measures, neglected children did not differ from nonmaltreated children on any of these measures over time (with SES and race controlled). Although the neglected group showed evidence of home adjustment problems at the time of the initial interviews (as Figure 11 shows), the difficulties had subsided enough by follow-up (see Table D) that the group did not differ when initial and follow-up data were combined for analysis.

On five of the nine socioemotional measures (self-concept, aggression, emotional adjustment, peer relationships, and delinquency), the raw scores of the neglected and comparison groups were nearly identical (see Figures 8, 9, 12, 13, and 14). Neglected children scored slightly worse on our measures of parent-reported problem behaviors and school adjustment problems, but the differences were not significant (see Figures 7 and 10).

Because of an unexpected racial disparity between our neglected group (81% white) and the abused (55%) and comparison (63%) groups, race was an important factor on one of our socioemotional measures–the Child Behavior Checklist Teacher Form. On this instrument, an apparent difference between the neglected and comparison groups (see Figure 6; Table C) was nullified because teachers reported a significantly higher number of behavior problems for white than black neglected children (this was true for abused children as well, but not for nonmaltreated children). Thus, with both SES and race controlled, the neglect group did not differ significantly from the comparison group–logically, if the group had included more blacks, fewer problems would have been reported.

However, it is noteworthy that white neglected children were judged by teachers to be as problematic as abused children (very problematic indeed). Since no other measure showed significant differences between white and black children (including the parallel Parent Form of the Child Behavior Checklist), it is difficult to interpret this anomaly. Nevertheless, the finding deserves attention from teachers, practitioners, and researchers.

CASE PROFILE #7– BEN: GROWING UP NEGLECTED

Ben, 13, lived with his mother, stepfather, and four brothers in a small stucco house on a busy highway. The parents had been charged with neglect three months before our study began. CPS had cited inadequacies in nearly every realm of child care, including hygiene, health care, nutrition, clothing, physical safety in the home, availability of utilities, supervision of children, and parental consistency.

Neither parent had completed high school, and both worked sporadically at minimum wage jobs. Our stress inventory revealed a chaotic situation for the family during the year prior to the first interview, including unemployment, decreased income, a jail sentence, involvement in a fight, the death of a close friend, problems related to alcohol or drugs, and sex difficulties. By follow-up, the situation had become even worse. Marital separation, moving, serious illness, and imprisonment were added to the list, and the children were now living with their mother in a run-down trailer surrounded by debris.

At the time of the first interviews, Ben, like most of our neglect sample, was faring well in most areas of socioemotional development and adaptive functioning, but poorly in academics. He scored lower than 99% of his peers on standardized tests of language and math skills, and he had been absent 31 days of the previous school year. He had repeated at least one grade and was currently performing far below his fifth-grade peers in every subject. His teacher reported that Ben was happy and behaved appropriately in school, but that he simply "can't do the work." Ben scored low on self-concept (he saw himself as nervous, clumsy, unpopular, and "dumb about most things"), and his teacher reported a fair number of behavior problems, depicting him as somewhat fearful and withdrawn. Otherwise, Ben seemed fairly well adjusted. He had many friends, and he had never been in trouble with juvenile authorities.

At follow-up, Ben had been promoted to the sixth grade, but his academic struggles were still apparent. His new teacher identified nearly twice the number of behavior problems as his 5th grade teacher, including: depressed, self-destructive, feels unloved, fearful, withdrawn, apathetic, overtired, and "talks about killing self." In contrast, both Ben and his mother reported few socioemotional problems for Ben at follow-up. Apparently, he was happy with his family; got along well with his mother, brothers, teachers, and peers; and had a much higher self-concept than the year before. Indeed, he scored some 20 points higher than before on the Piers-Harris. He no longer saw himself as shy, unhappy, nervous, worried, unpopular, picked on, hot-tempered, poorly behaved, or fearful.

These inconsistencies are puzzling. Was Ben doing as well at follow-up as he and his mother declared, or was the teacher's observation of serious signs of maladjustment correct? Although the CPS case on the family was still open, there had been no subsequent reports of neglect. Ben's mother reported that she was much happier than the year before, liked her new neighborhood much more than the old, and now spent more time with friends. She reported even fewer behavior problems for Ben (almost none) than she had the year before. At last report, however, Ben had dropped out of school despite "a lot of effort" by school personnel to keep him in, and he was reportedly receiving little supervision at home.

Ben's case largely fits the profile our research established for *white,* school-age, neglected children. They displayed a tendency to function poorly academically, normally on measures of socioemotional development *except* for teacher-reported problem behaviors, and normally in practical skills. The high stress levels in the family seem to have contributed to Ben's school problems.

DISCUSSION

We had expected to find academic delays in the school-age neglected children we studied, but the delays we found were far more severe than anticipated. These children scored *extremely* low on standardized tests and other indicators of school performance. Our finding of adaptive strengths in neglected children were unexpected but not startling. It makes sense that older neglected children would manage to pick up the skills they need for survival. On the other hand, the lack of social and emotional problems for school-age neglected children came as a total surprise. A large body of previous research has firmly established the negative socioemotional consequences of neglect for younger children. Our findings suggest that neglect in later childhood is less likely to interfere with socioemotional development than neglect at an earlier age.

According to CPS (Child Protective Services) records, two-thirds of our neglected sample had experienced only recent neglect. Interestingly, we found that children who were reported as chronically neglected did not function more poorly on any of our academic or socioemotional measures than those only recently neglected. It seems possible, even likely, that many of the children who were reported only recently may also have experienced undetected neglect earlier in their lives. Certainly the group's academic difficulties are not a recent development, but we can only speculate as to whether these neglected children may have overcome earlier socioemotional problems through maturation and the socialization opportunities available to older children. By the school-age years, socioemotional processes may be more open to modification by outside influences than are cognitive processes.[1]

Of course, it is possible that the lack of significant differences on socioemotional measures could be the result of testing bias. Both anecdotal and empirical evidence suggest that neglected children and their parents have difficulty in testing and interview situations, and that they give minimal, socially desirable responses to questions. We were aware of this potential problem, however, and employed only experienced interviewers who had attained at least master's degrees in the social sciences. These interviewers–blind to group identity–were able to establish sharp differences between abused and nonmaltreated children on all of our socioemotional measures.

Furthermore, teacher reports agreed with parent and child reports that the neglected group, as a whole, was doing socially and emotionally as well as the nonmaltreatment group. Additional evidence of the neglected children's social and emotional strengths came with our final updates. At last report, dropout rates for the neglected (21%) and abused (23%) groups were equivalent, but neglected children were less likely to be in juvenile justice facilities (0% vs. 9%) or to be teenage mothers (2% vs. 14%).

Thus, our results cannot easily be dismissed as chance outcomes. Nevertheless, our findings of initial problems in home adjustment for the neglected group, and in school behavior for the white neglected children, suggest that additional research is needed–particularly studies that utilize observation and outside sources to assess the school-age neglected child's socioemotional development.

Our research indicates that intervention with school-age neglected children should focus on improving school performance and attendance using approaches discussed in the previous chapter and Chapter Eight. Improvements in our neglected group's school performance at follow-up (after CPS services were provided to families) suggest that neglected school-age children respond positively to general intervention services. Theoretically, the provision of specific services for academic enhancement could boost neglected children's school progress dramatically. For school-age neglected children, approaches that capitalize on the child's socioemotional and adaptive competence should be emphasized (e.g., group teaching strategies, vocational classes).

CASE PROFILES #8– BRIEF UPDATES ON NEGLECT CASES

The following information was provided by CPS and/or school system personnel approximately two years after our final interviews. The information is spotty, and we have no updated information at all on 13 neglected children (27%; eight girls, five boys). (Note: The names given are fictitious.)

- Gunther (now 11) and his siblings were returned to the custody of their parents who "immediately left the state." There has been no further contact with the family by CPS or school personnel.
- Tilly (11) is a "C student" in sixth grade.
- Tasha (12) is working at grade level in fifth grade, but is frequently absent.
- Betsy (12) is working at grade level in the fifth grade, and she is described as a "good kid."
- Carrie (13) is doing "very well" in the fourth grade after being placed with her grandparents.
- Grant (13) is "doing fine" in the sixth grade, and he is in a gifted math class.
- Rhonda (13) is attending sixth grade and "has not missed a day of school this year."
- Curtis (14) is in a self-contained seventh-grade class for behavior disorders and is making good grades.
- William (14) is attending school (details unknown) and was recently placed in his grandmother's custody.

- Robert (14) and his siblings remain in foster care. CPS plans to initiate litigation to terminate parental rights and free Robert and his siblings for adoption. Robert is well adjusted but having academic problems in the sixth grade.
- Kate (14) is in the sixth grade. Attendance problems have diminished since she moved in with an aunt.
- Harry (14) is in a sixth-grade special education class and is working below grade level, although his attendance is satisfactory.
- Mary (15) is earning good grades in the eighth grade and "wants to be a lawyer."
- Christy (15; see Case Profile #10–Christy: In and Out of Foster Care) is in the eighth grade where she is "picked on" and has few friends. School personnel are aware of family arguments.
- Tommy (15) is "doing well" in the seventh grade. He is still in foster care.
- Selina (15) dropped out of school. Her whereabouts are unknown.
- Deanna (16) is in foster care and receives special education services for learning disabilities (grade level unknown).
- Larry (16) is in the ninth grade, but is frequently truant. He has been placed on probation by the juvenile justice system for truancy. There have been 13 new referrals for neglect.
- Ben (16; see Case Profile #7–Ben: Growing Up Neglected) dropped out of school and reportedly receives little supervision at home.
- Patty (16) has shown recent improvement and is in the eighth grade. Allegations of sexual abuse have been confirmed, and the family is involved in counseling.
- Nina (17) is performing satisfactorily in the ninth grade.
- Angela (17) is currently in the 11th grade. She has lived in a foster home since her mother died.
- Michael (17; see Case Profile #9–Michael: In Distress) is displaying problem behaviors at school (grade level unknown) and complains of frequent nightmares.
- Helena (17) is an average student in the ninth grade. She continues in foster care.

- Craig (17) is doing well in vocational classes.
- Alan (17) dropped out of school in the ninth grade and has become involved with the juvenile justice system. He is described as "belligerent." There have been recent reports of both abuse and neglect. (Note: Alan's family reported severe stress levels, especially at follow-up, including a period of homelessness.)
- Brian (18) dropped out of school in the eighth grade, and he is now working. He lives with the family of a friend.
- Linda (18) dropped out of school and disappeared. Her family moved to another state, and Linda "has never turned up either here or . . . with her family. At one point, the decomposed body of a young woman was found in ______ County. For a while, police suspected that it might be [Linda], but it turned out not to be."
- Ramona (18) was in a juvenile facility for delinquent behavior at the time of our follow-up interview. Since then, she has been placed in a girls' home, run away, dropped out of school, and become pregnant. (Note: Ramona has experienced multiple foster-care placements.)
- Susan (18) was in a group home out-of-county at the time of our follow-up interviews, but she was subsequently "discharged because of unruly behavior." She is currently living with her mother and is attending 10th-grade special education classes "on a regular basis."
- Stephanie (19) dropped out of school and is now married.
- Keith (19) dropped out of junior high at age 16 and is currently employed through Vocational Rehabilitation.
- Mary Ann (19) dropped out of school, married her foster brother, and has one child.
- Teresa (19) dropped out of school. Her whereabouts are unknown.

CONCLUSION

This chapter has presented a profile of the neglected school-age child. In sharp contrast to physically abused children, the neglected children we studied were faring well except in the classroom, where their academic deficits were severe. The next chapter will expand our profiles of maltreated children through discussion of family and background characteristics.

NOTE

1. J.L. Aber and D. Cicchetti, "The Socio-emotional Development of Maltreated Children," in *Theory and Research on Behavioral Pediatrics,* ed. B.M. Lester and M.W. Yogman (New York: Plenum Press, 1984), 147-205.

Chapter Six

Family and Background Characteristics of Abused and Neglected School-Age Children

The abused and neglected children we studied may have come to the attention of CPS (Child Protective Services) authorities because of a specific incident of maltreatment, but, in all likelihood, this incident represented the tip of the iceberg. The severe developmental deficits we found in maltreated children certainly did not result from a single act of abuse or neglect. More likely, these delays evolved gradually in response to ongoing patterns of family dysfunction. This chapter presents findings and implications relative to the family and background characteristics of the maltreated children we studied.

FAMILY PROBLEMS

Based on past research and theory, we expected the families of abused or neglected children to report more stress, parental depression, and social isolation than comparison families. The results only partly confirmed our expectations (see Table E, Appendix). The maltreating families did report extremely high levels of stress from life events. Next to maltreatment, family stress predicted children's poor functioning better than any other variable we examined (see Table 3, Chapter Three). Parental depression was evident for abuse group but not neglect group respondents. Surprisingly, social isolation, which has been strongly linked to maltreatment (especially neglect) by past research, was unrelated to abuse or neglect in our study.

CASE PROFILE #9– MICHAEL: IN DISTRESS

Michael was 13 when our study began. He was living with his divorced unemployed mother and his 19-year-old brother. A few months earlier, charges of neglect had been substantiated based on failure to provide Michael with needed health care, nutrition, clothing, and secure housing with needed utilities. The Life Events Inventory completed by Michael's mother revealed extreme levels of stress for the family during the past year (higher than for any other family we studied), including serious problems with unemployment, money, health, drugs/alcohol, legal authorities, accidents, suicide attempts, quarrels with neighbors, and family arguments. Similar stressors were reported at follow-up. Many of these problems may have involved Michael's 19-year-old brother, who was apparently in prison at follow-up.

Although Michael had never repeated a grade, he was an extremely poor student. He scored lower than 98% of his peers on standardized tests, and he earned mostly F's in his eighth-grade classes. He was frequently absent or tardy and "hated" school (but expected to graduate). Teachers reported an extremely high number of behavior problems for Michael, characterizing him as argumentative, defiant, fidgety, disobedient, disruptive, accident-prone, irritable, hot-tempered, and easily frustrated. One teacher noted that Michael spoke of Satanic ideas. Michael reported that he had been paddled and suspended from school many times. His mother also complained of excessive behavior problems at home, identifying Michael as restless, clinging, demanding, destructive, impulsive, high-strung, and poorly coordinated.

Unlike most of the maltreated children in our study, Michael was performing far below his peers in motor, personal care, and community/work skills. For example, he reportedly could not (at age 13) cut a straight line with scissors, eat soup without spilling, select clothing appropriate for the occasion, use a vacuum cleaner, or take a bus. The interviewer noted that during both interviews Michael showed no emotions, responded slowly, gave brief answers, and responded "I don't know" to many questions. However, his self-concept and self-reported feelings of aggression were in the normal range, and he had many friends (though he could think of no activities they engaged in other than "hanging out").

Michael's problems continued at follow-up, and by then he had become involved with the juvenile authorities for a delinquent offense. During the follow-up interview he admitted to skipping school, using drugs, stealing, hitting others, vandalizing property, and breaking and entering. At last report, Michael, at 16, was reportedly having severe behavior problems at school and frequent nightmares, and his mother had been diagnosed with a life-threatening illness.

Michael's situation is alarming. It is hard to imagine that he will graduate from high school or avoid serious problems with the authorities. With his marked socioemotional problems, he looks more like the abused children in our study than the neglected (though he lacks the practical skills of both groups). It seems plausible that the extreme stress in Michael's family contributed to his problems. Our study found stress to be the common thread for both types of maltreatment. Next to maltreatment itself, it was the strongest predictor of children's poor functioning–particularly poor school performance, problem behaviors, home maladjustment, peer maladjustment, and delinquency.

STRESS

Family stress has long been associated with child maltreatment, and our research extends this association to families of older abused or neglected children. Further, we were able to pinpoint specific stressors that may contribute to maltreatment of the school-age child. Both abusive and neglectful families in this study reported high levels of stress from a variety of life events that occurred during the year prior to the initial interviews. These ranged from quarrels with neighbors and extramarital affairs to jail sentences, "debt beyond means of repayment," and homelessness. Both types of maltreating families reported particularly high levels of stress related to alcohol or drug use by family members. Neglectful but not abusive families reported high levels of marital and interpersonal conflict. By follow-up, the neglectful group's stress levels had diminished somewhat (not significantly), but the abusive group's had not. Interestingly, with SES (socioeconomic status) controlled, the maltreating families did not report higher levels of unemployment, single parenthood, large family size, money troubles, legal troubles, bereavement, or family illness than nonmaltreating families.

There is no certainty that the identified stressors predated abuse or neglect in our sample. We asked about stressful events that occurred during the previous year, but abuse or neglect had occurred up to 18 months earlier. It is possible that being identified and treated by authorities as abusive or neglectful contributed to the substance abuse, marital and interpersonal problems, and other stressors for maltreating families. However, such problems usually evolve over time, and it is more likely that the elevated stress levels experienced by these families predated and contributed to abusive or neglectful parenting, as other researchers have suggested.

Not surprisingly, children from the most stressed families were functioning the most poorly on academic and socioemotional dimensions of development. Family stress was especially associated with academic difficulties, problem behavior in the home, maladjustment at home, peer relationship problems, and delinquency. It is difficult to disentangle the separate contributions of physical abuse and stress to abused children's poor functioning because stress and abuse have both been associated with childhood adjustment problems.[1] Future maltreatment research should probably control for family stress levels as well as SES.

PARENTAL DEPRESSION

Our finding that the abusive group's parents reported high levels of depression is not surprising; numerous studies have identified symptoms of depression in abusing parents. However, the relationship between depression and child abuse is far from clear. The literature on depression provides evidence that depressed mothers often relate to their children in a rejecting and hostile manner, and that they are more likely to use physical punishment than mothers who are not depressed.[2] Thus, it would seem that parental depression could lead to child abuse (especially when high levels of stress are present). However, those studies that assess parents only after abuse has been substantiated cannot determine if depression was present at the time of the abusive incident or if it occurred as a result of the family being identified by authorities as abusive. Nevertheless, our finding that the abusive group's parents reported no reduction in their depression at follow-up suggests that their despondency is chronic and deep-rooted.

Parental depression was particularly related to problem behaviors of the maltreated children we studied. This finding would be shaky if it relied only on parent reports, because depressed parents might be expected to consider their children troublesome, but teacher reports confirmed that the children of depressed parents displayed problem behaviors in the classroom as well. This consistency of results is rather intriguing given that parental depression was unrelated to any other dimension of socioemotional or academic development. Studies of the children of depressed but nonabusive parents have also linked children's problem behaviors with parental depression.[3] Thus, the connection appears to be strong. However, it is difficult to determine the dynamics involved–i.e., whether abuse, parental depression, or children's problem behaviors came first. Studies are needed to examine the sequence and processes involved.

SOCIAL ISOLATION

Social isolation from familial and community resources has long been seen as a precursor to maltreatment, especially neglect. In the present study, however, there were no significant differences among the groups in the level of support available or utilized from relatives, friends, neighbors, churches, or community agencies. It may be that these families of older maltreated children have had increased opportunities to establish social networks over the years. Or, given the limitations of our retrospective research design, it could be that social isolation existed at the time of the abusive or neglectful incidents but was ameliorated (perhaps through CPS efforts) before our first interviews took place. At any rate, at both initial and follow-up interviews, our two maltreatment groups reported levels of social support similar to those reported by nonmaltreating families.

THE ROLE OF SES

We know that low family SES exerts a profound negative influence on children's achievement and adjustment. Most of the families identified as physically abusive or neglectful come from the lower classes; thus the confounding effects of SES cannot be ignored in research on maltreated children. Studies often control for SES by using a comparison group that is matched to the maltreatment group(s) on such factors as income, education, and occupation. This procedure can rule out SES as an explanatory factor for group differences, but it does not allow clarification of the role SES plays in the various assessed dimensions of child development and family functioning. By using a representative comparison group and controlling for SES through statistical procedures, the present study allows us to look at the contribution of SES to child and family functioning.

In this study, low SES exerted a strong negative impact on children and families, with lower class children experiencing particular difficulties at school. Depressed scores on standardized tests, teachers' low assessments of performance, a high rate of absences and grade repeats, problem behaviors in the classroom, poor school adjustment, and low educational aspirations were all significantly related to poverty. Lower-class membership also predicted problem behaviors at home, aggression, delinquency, and maladjustment in every arena except peer relationships, where no class differences were found. Low SES children were more likely to appear in juvenile court, use drugs or alcohol, and report trouble controlling their tempers. On the other hand, sadness, suicidal tendencies, and sleep and appetite disturbances were unrelated to class. Most children, whether low or high SES, reported they were happy with their families and got along well with parents and friends (only the abused children reported problems in these areas).

There were overall differences on the Piers-Harris, with lower-class children reporting lower self-concept than children who were economically advantaged. It is notable that, although differences occurred on the Behavior, Intellectual, Anxiety, and Happiness and Satisfaction subscales, there were no differences on the Physical or Popularity subscales. Again, the latter reflected the lack of peer relationship problems for low SES children. On adaptive functioning measures, poor children were faring as well as their economically better-off peers on motor skills and personal care skills, but were lagging behind in community skills (time and punctuality, money and value, work skills, and home-community orientation).

Not surprisingly, lower-class families were more likely than their better-off counterparts to have experienced high levels of stress (especially stress from money troubles and alcohol or drug use by family members), unemployment, parental depression, and social isolation. Single parenthood and large family size were more common in these families. However, there were no reported class differences in levels of marital conflict.

It is apparent that there is substantial correlation between the factors associated with low SES and maltreatment in the present study. Since approximately two-thirds of the low SES families involved in the study were maltreating families, the differences attributed to low SES may instead reflect the impact of maltreatment. This would be especially true where both groups of maltreated children differed from nonmaltreated children. Thus, the poor school performance and high levels of family stress found for our low SES families could be due to the low scores on these measures by the two maltreatment groups. On the other hand, the lack of maltreatment effects on community skills and social support indicates that low SES is especially related to deficits in these areas. It is notable that physical abuse (and not neglect or low SES) is uniquely associated with problematic peer relationships.

THE EFFECTS OF RACE

The impact of race on outcome scores was of particular concern in the present study because of the unexpected racial disparity among our groups: our neglected group (81% white) was significantly more white than the abused (55%) and comparison (63%)

groups. Since a statewide breakdown of maltreatment subtypes by race was not available, we cannot be certain that these percentages reflect the racial distribution of abuse and neglect cases in Georgia. However, the CPS administrators and workers we queried agreed that most reported and substantiated neglect cases in the state involve white families. This is thought to reflect a dual standard for defining neglect in black and white families, with both reporting agents and CPS investigators considering white neglect more serious and black neglect more normative. Indeed, several administrators speculated that if consistent standards were applied, the system might well be inundated with black neglect cases.

Because of the significant racial differences among the groups, we implemented statistical controls to examine the separate contribution of race on outcome measures. There were few significant effects. With SES controlled, black children were slightly more likely than white children to display school performance deficits; low self-concept; problem behaviors at home; and problems with school adjustment, home adjustment, and emotional adjustment. They were slightly less likely to report elevated feelings of aggression. Black families reported slightly higher levels of parental depression, and white families were somewhat more likely to report high levels of stress from life events. None of these differences were statistically significant.

There were no racial differences in peer adjustment, delinquency, or marital conflict. However, we did find significant differences on our social support measure, with white families reporting less social support from kinship and community networks than black families. (This race effect did not change our finding that neglectful families are no more socially isolated than comparison families; indeed, if more black neglectful families had been included, social isolation would have been even less likely for the neglectful group as a whole.) Statistical controls for race changed the preliminary results of the study only for problem behavior in the classroom, where teachers reported that white neglected children displayed many more problems than black neglected children. This was true for abused children as well, but not for comparison children.

BACKGROUND CHARACTERISTICS

We expected that the most serious delays would occur in children who had experienced severe maltreatment, chronic maltreatment, multiple forms of maltreatment, sexual abuse, or foster care placement. However, there were few effects from these variables. Only the number of times (but not length of time) in foster care consistently predicted poor outcomes (see Table 3 in Chapter Three).

Severity of Maltreatment

There was not enough variation in the reported injuries from physical abuse to test for the effect of severity of abuse; few of the abused children had sustained injuries serious enough to require hospitalization (e.g., fractures, internal injuries). There was a much wider variation in the severity of neglect among neglectful families, but this factor was not predictive of poor functioning on any of our outcome measures. Children who were grossly neglected were doing as well as children who were only moderately neglected. This surprising result adds strength to our finding that the consequences of neglect for the school-age child are less pervasive than might be expected. The greater resources and autonomy of the older child may moderate the effects of neglect–even gross neglect–by caretakers.

To arrive at our severity of neglect scores, we used caseworker ratings of each maltreating family's provision of needed health care, nutrition, clothing, hygiene, housing, and supervision for their children. As expected, the neglectful families scored significantly more poorly than the abusive families. Additionally, our interviewers assessed each family (abusive, neglectful, nonmaltreating) in terms of household furnishings, sanitation, and safety factors. Their ratings were also as expected, with neglectful families scoring lowest, comparison families highest, and abusive families in between (see Table E). These results provide evidence of the validity of our participant groupings.

On the other hand, our control measure for parental aggression, the Conflict Tactics Scale, was unable to differentiate between abusive and nonabusive families (see Table E). Abusive group parents did not report using more physical aggression against their children than neglectful or comparison group parents. However, this result may reflect less on the validity of the measure than on group composition: the majority (68%) of the abusive group parent respondents were not the identified perpetrators of abuse in the family. Interestingly, abusive group parents did report that the abused children directed considerable aggression towards *them*–much more than neglectful or comparison group parents reported for their children. This provides yet another indicator of high aggression levels in the abused children.

Chronicity of Maltreatment

The majority of maltreated children had only experienced substantiated abuse or neglect within the previous 18 months, but others had long CPS histories. We found that children whose maltreatment could be considered chronic did not fare more poorly on any of our outcome measures than those who had only recently been maltreated. In fact, the only significant finding from this set of analyses ran contrary to our hypothesis: children who had experienced only recent maltreatment were more likely to display behavior problems at school than chronically maltreated children. Although it does make sense that children might react to new abuse or neglect with an increase in school behavior problems, it would be unreasonable to attach too much significance to this isolated finding. The overall lack of difference between recently and chronically maltreated children is of greater significance, and could indicate that chronic maltreatment was more prevalent in our sample than the records showed.

Multiple Forms of Maltreatment

According to caseworkers, 55% of the abused children in our sample (and 17% of the neglected) had experienced more than one form of maltreatment (i.e., physical abuse, neglect, sexual abuse) over the course of their CPS involvement. However, these children showed no effects from additional forms of maltreatment except on our delinquency scale, where a higher number of maltreatment subtypes predicted delinquent behavior.

Six of the maltreated children we studied had been both abused and neglected during the previous 18-month period. In each of these cases, physical abuse was considered the primary maltreatment classification. Thus, these children were placed in the abuse group for this study. Later analysis supported this classification decision: the breakdown of outcome scores showed that the children who had been both abused and neglected fit with the children who had been only abused, but differed from those who had been only neglected. Like their abused-only counterparts, these abused-neglected children were functioning more poorly than comparison children on all of our socioemotional measures as well as on overall school performance.

Sexual Abuse

Of the maltreated children we studied, 23% had been sexually abused at some time, including 32% of the abused group (7 girls) and 15% of the neglected group (4 girls; 3 boys). Mirroring our findings on multiple forms of maltreatment, we found no effect from sexual abuse except on our delinquency measure. This finding is undoubtedly age related: the oldest children were more likely both to have been sexually abused and to have engaged in delinquent behaviors. It may seem surprising that sexual abuse was unrelated to scores on other outcome measures, but the literature on sexual abuse does suggest that effects, though enduring, may be subtle and difficult to detect.[4]

Foster Care Placement

Nearly 29% (abused = 23%; neglected = 32%) of the maltreated children had been in foster care at some time. Studies have presented conflicting evidence as to whether maltreated children fare better when they are maintained in their own homes or placed in foster care settings. Our findings suggest that, although foster care placement per se may not be detrimental to children, a history of multiple placements is associated with socioemotional maladjustment. In this study, increases in the number of times a child had been placed in foster care were related to low self-concept, high levels of aggression, poor home adjustment, and poor emotional adjustment. Thus, it would appear that the effects of maltreatment are exacerbated by multiple placements. However, it cannot be determined from the present study whether multiple placements contributed to children's maladjustment or children's maladjustment led to multiple placements. In any case, special care should be given to assure the placement success of all children, especially those who show signs of maladjustment.

CASE PROFILE #10– CHRISTY: IN AND OUT OF FOSTER CARE

Twelve-year-old Christy had been placed in foster care for the third time in five years because of neglect by her natural parents. The most recent neglect charge involved serious parental inadequacies which included leaving Christy and her younger brother alone for extended periods of time and failing to provide basic and essential items of clothing for the children. Christy's academic performance was extremely poor. She tested lower than 95% of her peers in both language and math skills, and she had missed 25 days of the previous school year (prior to placement). She had repeated first and third grades and was now in the fifth grade; however, she said she liked school and expected to graduate. Her teacher reported few behavior problems for Christy, but noted that she was much less happy than most students.

Christy's foster mother described a significant amount of problem behavior in the home, including acting "too young for her age," bragging, clinging, day-dreaming, becoming "easily jealous," and being "too concerned with neatness or cleanliness." Christy reported that she was happy in her foster family, but that she had been decidedly unhappy in her natural family. She said she got along poorly with both parents who were unloving and "too restrictive." She reported many fears and worries, was sad nearly every day, and worried that terrible things would happen to her. She also had low self-concept, frequent nightmares and headaches, and a high level of aggressive feelings. She had thought about killing herself "once or twice" in the past six months. However, Christy seemed well adjusted in school and with peers, showed no evidence of delinquent behavior, and was functioning normally in terms of motor, self-care, and community skills.

The next year, Christy was back with her mother, who completed the follow-up interview. Christy's mother reported a high level of stressful life events during the preceding year (while Christy was in foster care), including a jail term, "debt beyond means of repayment," and a period of homelessness. She eventually found a job in a factory, moved into an apartment, and divorced her husband. Christy was returned home, but her younger brother was apparently still in placement at the time of our follow-up interviews. At this point the family seemed to have adequate social support, but Christy's mother was markedly depressed and hated the neighborhood where they lived.

Despite all the turmoil, including a change of schools, Christy showed improvement on nearly all of our academic and socioemotional measures at follow-up. Her grades and test scores increased, and her problem behaviors, fears, worries, and nightmares decreased. Whereas the year before she had hoped only to graduate from high school, she now aspired to a college degree. She reported that she got along well with her mother now, and she never thought of hurting herself. Her self-concept had also improved: the previous year she had described herself as unhappy, dumb, unlucky, and "picked on," but at follow-up she reported being happy, smart, lucky, and "an important member of my family." She did, however, report more feelings of aggression than in the previous year.

Christy's academic difficulties and improvement over time were characteristic of the neglected children we studied, but her socioemotional difficulties were not. Indeed, one of our most provocative findings was the lack of such problems among school-age neglected children. On the other hand, those children who, like Christy, had experienced multiple foster care placements had similar problems with low self-concept, elevated aggression, emotional maladjustment, and maladjustment at home. Thus, our findings could indicate that

Christy's socioemotional problems were particularly related to her multiple placements.

At latest report Christy, now 15, still lives with her mother and is still in school (eighth grade), but she is reportedly "picked on" by other students and has few friends. School personnel are aware of family arguments. We certainly hope that Christy will not require yet another placement. Treatment and supportive services seem essential if this outcome is to be avoided.

FOLLOW-UP CPS STATUS

Information provided by caseworkers revealed that 16 of the 22 abuse cases (73%) and 30 of the 47 neglect cases (65%) remained open at follow-up (6-12 months after the initial interviews). New reports of maltreatment had been substantiated for nine (41%) of the abused and seven (15%) of the neglected children. Three (14%) of the abused and one (2%) of the neglected children had been removed from their homes and placed in foster or institutional care; one (2%) neglected child had been returned home from foster placement; two (9%) abused children were living on their own at follow-up. Nine of the abused (41%) and 18 (39%) of the neglected children had moved to a new address by follow-up, compared with 13 (19%) of the comparison children. These data suggest that, although both groups of maltreated children displayed modest overall improvement on most outcome measures at follow-up, home situations continued to be unstable.

CONCLUSION AND IMPLICATIONS

Our findings regarding family and background factors have important implications for working with maltreated school-age children and their families. The data indicate that stress is a significant factor for child abuse and neglect, and that stressful conditions in the home contribute to children's negative functioning on academic and socioemotional measures. Thus, intervention with abusive and neglectful families should focus efforts on evaluating and alleviating family stress through concrete and therapeutic services.

Family-based services should include assistance with finances, housing, jobs, transportation, parenting skills, and other basic necessities. Efforts to improve parents' coping skills through relaxation, stress management, and cognitive self-control strategies may also be beneficial.[5] Both parents and children from the most stressed families could benefit from therapy to address socioemotional problems, and the children are likely to need academic remediation. Special attention should be given to diagnosing and treating substance abuse problems in maltreating families. Alcohol and drug counselors should be trained to identify and report maltreatment situations involving their clients.

In this study, abusive and neglectful families of school-age children differed in several respects. The high levels of marital conflict we found in neglectful families suggest that couples or family therapy would be useful for these families; indeed, family therapy has proven particularly effective with families involved in child neglect.[6] In abuse cases, parents should be evaluated for depressive symptomatology, and then offered appropriate treatment services. When parental depression is identified, special attention should be focused on assessing and treating child behavior problems in school and at home.

Among the most surprising findings was the general lack of effect found for specific background factors in the children's maltreatment histories. It made little difference whether maltreatment was severe or only moderate, chronic or only recent, multiform or singular; whether sexual abuse was involved; or whether the child had spent years or only days in foster care–the abuse or neglect classification alone was the determining factor for child functioning. These surprising results suggest that intervention efforts with maltreated school-age children should focus primarily on recent physical abuse or neglect incidents. Of the background variables we examined, only multiple foster care placements were consistently related to poor functioning. Therapeutic services should be provided for all children placed in foster care, but particularly for those experiencing re-placement or socioemotional problems.

This chapter has examined the role of family and background

factors in the maltreatment of school-age children. The next chapter will explore current system realities that hinder the delivery of needed services to maltreated children and their families.

NOTES

1. B.E. Compas, "Stress and Life Events During Childhood and Adolescence," *Clinical Psychology Review* 7 (1987): 275-302.

2. M.M. Weissman and E.S. Paykel, *The Depressed Woman: A Study of Social Relationships* (Chicago: University of Chicago Press, 1974); D. Belle, ed., *Lives in Stress: Women and Depression* (Beverly Hills: Sage, 1982).

3. S. Wolff, "Social and Family Background of Preschool Children with Behaviour Disorders Attending a Child Guidance Clinic," *Journal of Child Psychology and Psychiatry* 2 (1961): 260-8; N. Richman, "Depression in Mothers of Preschool Children," *Journal of Child Psychology and Psychiatry* 17 (1976): 75-78.

4. A. Browne and D. Finkelhor, "Impact of Child Sexual Abuse: A Review of the Research," *Psychological Bulletin* 99 (1986): 66-77.

5. S. Ambrose, A. Hazzard, and J. Haworth, "Cognitive Behavioral Parenting Groups for Abusive Families," *Child Abuse and Neglect* 4 (1980): 119-24; C. Koverola, D. Elliott-Faust, and D. Wolfe, "Clinical Issues in the Behavioral Treatment of a Child Abusive Mother Experiencing Multiple Life Stresses," *Journal of Clinical Child Psychology* 13 (1984): 187-91.

6. D. Daro, *Confronting Child Abuse: Research for Effective Program Design* (New York: Free Press, 1988).

Chapter Seven

Societal Responses to Child Maltreatment

Twenty years ago, there were few laws specifically pertaining to child abuse and neglect. Now, child maltreatment has come to be regarded as a major social problem requiring extensive state involvement. As the prevalence and negative consequences of child maltreatment became more widely known, state and federal laws continuously broadened the legal grounds for intervention. Additionally, various agencies developed strategies for dealing with the problem.

There can be no doubt that intervention efforts have saved lives and benefited thousands of children. Nevertheless, societal response to child maltreatment has been rapidly evolving at a time of severe funding constraints, and services have not kept pace with the huge increase in reported cases. The fact is that it is simply not possible to serve every case adequately without many more resources. Indeed, the U.S. Advisory Board on Child Abuse and Neglect recently declared a "national emergency" in child protection.[1]

Children (especially poor children) have rarely been a priority for our elected officials or the voting populace. Budgetary cutbacks in the past decade have been especially hard on social programs for children and families. As this chapter will show, funding limitations and a lack of leadership have led to a highly fragmented service delivery system for maltreated children. This system is characterized by "turf" issues and narrow treatment policies that focus on symptoms rather than family systems and processes. The older maltreated child is particularly likely to be underserved or misserved by the overburdened agencies within the system. The older the child gets, the more likely it is that he or she will receive inappropriate (sometimes grossly inappropriate) treatment by service agencies.

Although we did not examine the specific interventions used in cases we studied, the services provided undoubtedly fell into the usual array of services offered in Georgia, the South, and many other parts of the country. This chapter gives an overview of the policies and practices that have evolved, both here and elsewhere (and under severe funding constraints almost everywhere), for dealing with the older maltreated child. Although our analysis is highly critical of current policies and practices, our comments are in no way intended to disparage front-line workers. The CPS (Child Protective Services) and school personnel with whom we worked closely, and the juvenile justice and mental health personnel whom we consulted, were (almost without exception) extraordinarily dedicated, caring, and resourceful workers who were doing the best they could with the limited resources and training at hand.

CPS AGENCIES

Almost all communities now have CPS agencies to receive reports of abuse and neglect, investigate these reports, and determine whether protective measures and treatment services are needed. In serious cases, caseworkers may immediately remove a child from the home on an emergency basis. More often, services are offered to parents on a voluntary basis. These services may include financial assistance, counseling, homemaker assistance, parenting classes, support groups, and advocacy on behalf of the family with landlords, police, schools, and other agencies. However, the threat of court action is always present. If the parents refuse to accept the agency's planned services, the services may be imposed by the court, or CPS may be given custody so the child can be placed in foster care.

The caseworkers handling these tasks carry an awesome responsibility. Indeed, it is a dual responsibility–in most cases, the same worker is charged with both investigating the reported maltreatment and providing immediate and long-term services to the family. To protect the child from further harm while simultaneously establishing a therapeutic relationship with the family, caseworkers must juggle the inherently conflicting roles of control agent and social worker. The job would be difficult under the best of circumstances, but its difficulty is immensely compounded by staffing and funding limitations.

Across the country, increases in reports of abuse and neglect have far outstripped increases in CPS staff. A number of states have even reduced staff in the face of federal cutbacks.[2] As a result, time and resources are increasingly spent on investigating more and more reports rather than on providing services to families who need them. Determining a family's specific needs and providing or locating appropriate services are time-consuming tasks. Not surprisingly, studies have found that the majority of families are not receiving crucial and timely services to prevent either the recurrence of maltreatment or the placement of children in foster care.[3]

In fully half of all cases, the maltreatment continues after CPS becomes involved.[4] And, as reports have increased, the substantiation rate has dropped–from 65% in 1975[5] to 35% in recent years.[6] Because of funding constraints, only the most serious cases can be added to caseloads; many of the unsubstantiated cases are likely to be re-reported, perhaps this time with more severe injury to the child.[7]

CPS agencies are simply overwhelmed. Low pay, long hours, large caseloads, insufficient training and supervision, burnout, and the threat of malpractice lawsuits all contribute to a high turnover rate in CPS offices (turnover of 50% a year is not uncommon in some Georgia offices). Social workers have abandoned child welfare in droves. Hiring standards have steadily eroded, and the field has been largely deprofessionalized. In Georgia, CPS workers have completed an *average* of only 16 years of education, and degrees need not be in social work or related fields.[8] Once hired, these workers are given one to two weeks of training, caseloads averaging 34 families (the Child Welfare League recommends 17), and starting salaries of $20,000.[9] From this meager base they are sent out to make unannounced visits to unstable families in crisis, judge whether children are in imminent danger or can safely remain in the home, and decide which of the few services at their disposal should be provided.

The high turnover rate and low hiring standards put children and families at risk through inadequate protective measures, gaps and delays in services, and poor decision making. CPS agencies across the nation report that staff-related problems are the principal barrier to the provision of appropriate services.[10] With frequent staff changes, more and more decisions are based on the written record rather than the memory and knowledge of caseworkers who have had live contact with the child and family. Further, a high turnover of caseworkers makes it more likely that children will be subjected to multiple placements,[11] which our study found to be particularly detrimental to children's well-being. And, in maltreatment cases, *not* making a decision may have an effect as powerful as making a decision (for example, when an emergency placement is left in place because of staff shortages).

Federal legislation has exacerbated the problems by increasing paperwork requirements while curtailing funding for family support services. The high levels of stress reported by the maltreating families in our study (and many others) suggest that intervention efforts ought to focus on relieving the pressures these families face. State CPS agencies have advised the U.S. Congress that federal funds should be shifted or added to support more treatment and prevention efforts.[12] But despite lip service in the halls of Congress to the ideal of family preservation, federal funding mechanisms provide strong incentives for workers to remove more and more children from their homes. While out-of-home placements are reimbursed through an open-ended entitlement program (the authorization level is "such funds as are necessary"), federal funds for services that could prevent placement have not yet reached even the scanty level authorized in 1980.[13]

Dramatic increases in foster care placements are occurring nationwide: there are now nearly 400,000 foster children in the United States. Between 1985 and 1988, the number of children entering foster care increased by 27%, and children are staying in placement longer and experiencing more repeat placements.[14] In Georgia, the foster care population rose 44% between 1984 and 1988.[15] These increases have occurred despite estimates that maintaining a child in foster care is nearly five times as costly as providing support services to maintain that child in his or her own home.[16] The staggering cost of placement for hundreds of thousands of children has begun to alarm federal officials; so far, their response has been ambiguous. Although fiscal policies favor placement, federal reimbursement for foster care payments already paid out by states are often held up, sometimes for years.[17] The delays place a heavy fiscal burden on states.

There are many indications that the quality of care provided to foster children is slipping badly–too often, children are placed in homes that are no better or even worse than their own homes. Agencies are losing established foster families because essential supports are not provided. One study of a large Midwestern foster care system found that 97% of the foster parents had received no foster parent training, some 90% had had no recorded contact with caseworkers in the previous year, and 14% were suspected of abusing or neglecting the foster children in their care.[18] Recruitment of adequate foster parents has become exceedingly difficult. Agencies have not adapted to new demographic realities, and, they continue to screen out single parents and families in which both parents work. Highly qualified applicants who are willing to take in one foster child are screened out because staff shortages dictate the placement of more children in fewer homes (it takes less time to visit five children in one home than the same five in different homes).

With the pool of foster families drying up, "temporary" emergency shelters are increasingly being used as more permanent placements. The 22 shelters in Georgia are horrendously overcrowded, with two or three babies sharing a crib at times, and older children sleeping on the floor.[19] Surely, if the state exercises its power to "protect" children from maltreatment by their families, it is obligated to ensure their safety and well-being in alternate placements.

Once a child is placed, it is all too easy to put the case on a back burner. Although federal legislation requires periodic review of foster care cases, the guidelines are vague and hearings are generally brief and perfunctory.[20] Staff and resource shortages often prevent working with the natural parents toward family reunification. While in foster care, children rarely receive adequate treatment for their emotional and developmental problems,[21] and adolescents are not adequately prepared for independent living.[22] Only a tiny percentage of foster children are ever freed for adoption because legal procedures to terminate parental rights are complex and time-consuming.[23]

The lack of staff and resources works especially against the older child. Most older children served by CPS are those who have been sexually abused. Physically abused or neglected older children and their families are much less likely to be added to caseloads. They may instead be referred to other systems, especially juvenile justice and mental health. CPS agencies are ill-equipped to manage or place acting-out children and adolescents. Caseworkers are often unfamiliar with research on latency-age and adolescent development, and they may believe that older children are less likely to be harmed by parental mistreatment. Even when cases *are* opened on older children, the children themselves are unlikely to receive needed treatment. Since most CPS agencies are mandated to work with maltreating parents but not with the maltreated child, funding constraints generally preclude providing direct services to children.

The failure of the child welfare system to provide effective services undoubtedly leads to underreporting of abused and neglected children. Although reporting rates have increased steadily, there is evidence that professionals (e.g., teachers, social workers, physicians, nurses, child care workers, and juvenile justice workers) still report fewer than 50% of maltreatment cases known to them. This goes on despite strict reporting laws that hold them liable for not reporting and offer them immunity from civil suit if they do report.[24] Many professionals may not report endangered children because they are afraid of bringing further harm to the child.

There is evidence that the majority of unreported cases involve school-age maltreated children.[25] Our research indicates that these children need help and that many do show modest improvement after CPS involvement. Thus, all suspected cases of abuse or neglect ought to be reported. However, professional hesitancy to report will surely persist until the recognized shortcomings of the CPS system are addressed.

THE JUVENILE JUSTICE SYSTEM

Although child abuse and neglect are punishable as crimes in some states, few cases are prosecuted in criminal court because the process is time-consuming and difficult, the case may be lost, and the imprisonment of the perpetrator does not usually resolve the family's problems. Instead, physical abuse and neglect cases are generally heard by juvenile or family courts, which operate under less stringent civil law guidelines. In theory, these courts offer greater flexibility for judges to determine and promote the best interests of the child. In practice, however, funding constraints of the justice system parallel those in CPS, and the courts are so clogged with cases that they cannot begin to give a fair hearing to each one. In large urban areas, one judge may hear as many as 100 abuse and neglect cases per day.[26] A hearing to determine whether a child will be removed from the home may last less than five minutes.

Judges assigned to juvenile and family courts are often those with the least seniority and experience. In many jurisdictions, judges are rotated in and out of juvenile and family court positions every three to six months.[27] Because few judges are adequately trained in child welfare issues, decisions rely heavily on the conclusory recommendations of overburdened caseworkers and may occasionally reflect a judge's personal bias. Although federal law mandates that any state receiving federal funds for child abuse and neglect must provide independent representation (a guardian ad litem) for all child victims in courtroom proceedings, the law is not enforced. In Georgia, three fourths of judges surveyed by telephone were not even aware of the law.[28]

CASE PROFILE #11– SARA: WHEN THE SYSTEM FAILS

Fourteen-year-old Sara lived with her mother and stepfather, both of whom worked in blue-collar jobs. The family had moved to the area the previous year and had purchased a house a few miles outside of town. According to CPS, Sara had been physically abused by her stepfather eight months before the study began. She had also been sexually abused by an uncle and by her mother's former live-in boyfriend several years earlier. The caseworker found no evidence of neglect; the family apparently provided amply for Sara's physical needs.

Sara's mother reported a high number of stressors for the previous year, including moving, quarrels with neighbors, a substantial decrease in income, the death of a close friend, prolonged ill health, and problems with children (Sara's 16-year-old brother had apparently been placed in a juvenile facility). However, there were no indications of parental depression, and the family's support network seemed adequate.

At the time of the first interviews, Sara liked school "a lot" and was rarely absent, but was performing far below grade level. She had repeated several grades, was now two years older than most of her sixth-grade classmates, and did not expect to graduate. No standardized test scores were available from her previous school, but both teacher respondents noted that Sara could do good work "when she does any." Her teachers reported a high number of behavior problems in school, including nervousness, distractibility, daydreaming, inability to concentrate, failure to complete assignments, and talking too much.

Her mother reported a similar array of behavior problems at home, but Sara seemed well adjusted in other respects. She saw herself as smart, happy, and popular; acknowledged few feelings of aggression; had never been in trouble with the law; and scored high on all dimensions of adaptive functioning. She claimed to have 50 good friends, few fears or worries, and no somatic problems. Thus, despite her academic and behavioral problems, Sara was faring better than most of the abused children in our study.

By follow-up, however, there had been new reports of physical abuse, and Sara had been placed in a group home in a different county. After considerable effort, we were able to obtain agreement from her new school and houseparents to conduct our follow-up procedures. However, a few days before the interviews were scheduled to take place, Sara appeared in court for a custody hearing. The judge, acting against CPS recommendations, awarded custody to her natural father who lived in another state. Sara, now 15, immediately left Georgia with her father. Two days later she was married to her father's middle-aged best friend.

The ill-considered decision to place Sara in her father's custody likely reflects the juvenile court's lack of time, resources, and training as well as the failure to provide independent representation as required by law.

All these factors work against ensuring the best interests of the child in maltreatment cases; however, the older maltreated child is at special risk from the juvenile justice system. As our study documented, older abused children typically display high levels of disturbed, aggressive, and delinquent behavior. When these children reach their teens, their status as victims may be increasingly overlooked. They may be inappropriately referred to juvenile authorities for offenses that should be considered of secondary importance to the parental maltreatment. Research indicates that between 40 and 90 percent of children who are charged with offenses have been maltreated.[29] Yet, no consistent policy has been established at the federal or state level for dealing with these youth. Written policy guidelines are generally not available to staff at any level of the juvenile justice system.[30]

Runaways, who may be attempting to avoid an abusive or neglectful environment, are typically adjudicated as status offenders (a "status offense" is a juvenile transgression which would not be considered an offense if committed by an adult). Studies suggest that many, perhaps the majority, of runaways are running from abusive homes.[31] Those youth who act out often are labeled delinquent in spite of case history material showing parental mistreatment. Police and juvenile authorities generally accept the parents' position that the child is the problem. Law enforcement officers in particular place great emphasis on the older child's demeanor. They may refer a case to the justice system rather than CPS because they do not look beyond the child's "attitude."

Once adjudicated, these children are either returned to their maltreating family environments or placed in institutional settings (Youth Development Centers in Georgia) where, because of overcrowding and low standards, they may be subjected to further abuse by other inmates or staff.[32] Research shows that juvenile offenders with a history of maltreatment are more likely than nonmaltreated offenders to be placed in institutions,[33] and they spend almost twice as much time in the system.[34]

Some juvenile justice agencies have established their own version of foster care (called Attention Homes or contract homes in Georgia) where rules are strict and punishment may be harsh. (In the opinion of one caseworker who participated in our study, the disciplinary measures used in contract homes in her community verged on abuse.)

Discussions with Georgia police officials, juvenile authorities, and judges paint a bleak picture of the system. The lack of services in many communities leads to a revolving door phenomenon: the same children enter the system repeatedly, sinking deeper and deeper into a deviant lifestyle until they can be transferred to an adult court. Everyone knows the problems stem from deplorable home environments, but the focus must remain on the child because resources are severely limited. One judge acknowledged that he sometimes commits a child to institutional or contract home placement primarily to remove the child from a bad home environment. The cases are not referred to CPS because "there aren't enough foster homes to go around."

Although some communities provide innovative programs for juvenile offenders and their families, few funds are available through the juvenile justice system for family-based intervention and prevention efforts. While the number of youth in juvenile facilities has increased dramatically (27% from 1979 to 1987; from 71,922 to 91,646), funding for the federal Office of Juvenile Justice and Delinquency Prevention has dropped by one third over the past decade.[35] Because of the juvenile justice system's narrow focus on the child's problematic behavior, the underlying family problems are not resolved, younger siblings may be left at risk, and the institutionalized youth may become locked into a deviant lifestyle.

THE MENTAL HEALTH SYSTEM

There is an implicit assumption that stopping the abuse or neglect will resolve the child's problems; however, protection from future maltreatment does not guarantee that psychological scars will vanish. (Indeed, if protection entails placement in foster care, the child is likely to experience additional distress.) The overwhelming problems of the abused children in our study certainly call out for therapeutic intervention, and there is every indication that such intervention would help. Research shows that maltreated children do respond positively to both individual and group therapy. These therapies have been proven to effectively alleviate psychological problems as well as reduce the likelihood that maltreatment will recur.[36] However, at present, maltreated children are unlikely to receive mental health services.

Federal funds for mental health programs dropped precipitously in the 1980s. Targeted funds for a range of child and adolescent mental health services were eliminated entirely in 1981. Currently, only 10% of federal mental health funds are earmarked for disturbed children and youth, though children and youth comprise approximately one third of the population. Medicaid, the medical service program for low-income families, provides very limited coverage for outpatient mental health services. Private insurers have sharply reduced their payments for such services as well. State funds for children's services are notoriously meager–many of Georgia's community mental health centers have no children's specialists at all.

Currently, only the most seriously disturbed children get help; thus, more funds are going for residential treatment than outpatient services. The number of children placed in mental health inpatient facilities increased 60% between 1983 and 1987 (from 34,000 to over 54,000).[37] It appears that out-of-home placements are becoming the primary "service" provided to children by CPS, juvenile justice, and mental health agencies.

There are no estimates of how many children in mental health facilities have been abused or neglected by parents, but the number is probably substantial. In some respects, these children may be luckier than those who come to the attention of the juvenile justice system because they may receive more sympathetic treatment. However, institutionalization in any form is extremely disruptive to children, and it may involve inhumane or inadequate treatment. For a child committed to a mental health facility, the length of stay may be indefinite (perhaps years), and the child is given a diagnostic label that may have stigmatizing effects far into the future. Further, if the child is the focus of intervention rather than the family, the maltreatment may never be addressed.

SCHOOLS

Our study found that the problems of older abused or neglected children are particularly apparent in the school environment, yet the role of the schools in dealing with maltreated children is rarely discussed. Due to their unique position in our communities, schools should be a central focus of intervention efforts, but this has not occurred. Although schools have played an important role in identifying and reporting suspected cases of child abuse and neglect, it is a sad fact that the problems of maltreated children are often exacerbated by our educational system. Administrators are increasingly focusing on standardized test scores and discipline, and arguing that other problems should be addressed by other agencies.

Maltreated children, however, do not leave their problems at the schoolhouse door. Many of these children are underachieving, difficult students for whom school may be a very negative experience. Most schools simply do not have the resources to adequately meet the special needs of these children. Typically, low achieving students are "socially promoted" until they are old enough to drop out; disruptive students are paddled, suspended, or expelled. The rules and regulations, geared for normal children, are ritualistically enforced despite individual differences and needs.

School discipline has become a major issue everywhere, and many educators now feel as if they are under siege. As families and communities deteriorate, the schools must deal with increasing numbers of "problem" students. Funding limitations and societal expectations have produced schools that focus heavily on maintaining high levels of control. In the face of budget cuts, support services (e.g., school social workers and counselors) are often the first to go. That leaves overburdened administrators, teachers, and office secretaries to handle the problems. Working under severe role pressures, these authority figures tend to respond to crises in a reflexive, punishment-oriented manner. For the acting-out child from an abusive family, episodes at school may fit a familiar pattern of provocative behavior met by coercive authority. Above all, what this child needs is a supportive environment where reasonable rules are fairly and consistently enforced, and where adults view crises as opportunities to model and teach effective coping skills.

These days, many students with special needs are apt to be "mainstreamed" rather than provided with special classes. This is especially true for students who are socioemotionally impaired (SEI), though these children are particularly problematic in the regular classroom.[38] In a large class, the presence of one or two disturbed students is likely to disrupt learning for the entire class. The disruptive student may experience rejection by teachers and other students. If this child comes from a maltreating environment, feelings of alienation that began in the home may extend to the school and to society in general, with disastrous consequences.

As recently as two decades ago, several national commissions argued that a child's success in school depended primarily on genetic factors and qualities of the home environment.[39] Differences in such factors as school budgets, class sizes, curriculum, and teacher characteristics were thought to have little or no impact on student success rates. Recent studies refute these assumptions.[40] Michael Rutter and his associates found that well-run schools in disadvantaged communities had a positive effect, not only on academic achievement, but also on problem behaviors and on rates of truancy, dropping out, and delinquency. The most successful schools had a startling impact on students.

We already know much of what needs to be done. The recommendations given in the next chapter are not revolutionary ideas. They have already been successfully implemented in many progressive school systems to enhance the potential of all students. The results of our study suggest that school functioning is the most damaged aspect of development for maltreated school-age children. For these children, educational reforms could make the difference, not only at school but in the larger society.

LACK OF INTERAGENCY COORDINATION

Older maltreated children are likely to be multiproblem children who require a multidisciplinary intervention approach. However, the systems that serve children focus on single problems such as abuse and neglect, delinquency, emotional problems, running away, or school behavior or performance problems. In most communities, interagency coordination of services and goals is almost nonexistent, yet it seems a matter of chance whether a child will end up in CPS, juvenile justice, mental health, or some other service agency. In fact, no system wants to claim the older multiproblem child. Because of the shortage of resources in all systems, agencies battle to avoid taking primary responsibility for an older child, especially since intervention so often involves expensive out-of-home care. Older children are hard to place, unlikely to be adopted, and may require long-term care because their family situations often prove intractible, especially with so few family-based services available.

Shortages and inappropriate services are common in all the systems, and many older multiproblem children are underserved or not served at all. An abused child's problems may not receive attention (despite a troubled school career and obvious signs of dysfunction) until a crisis is at hand. If one symptom does not elicit help, others may appear; or dysfunctional behaviors may escalate until someone finally does pay attention. By this time, the child may not look much like a victim, and he or she may be labeled as delinquent, a status offender, a drug addict, a runaway, or emotionally disturbed rather than abused. These labels reflect agency orientations more than the actual problems of the child and family. Indeed, labels are sometimes adjusted across systems to fit available (or unavailable) services.[41] (Thus, there *is* interagency coordination, but it consists of hidden practices which circumvent both public scrutiny and accountability to the community.)

Whichever system a child enters, there is an increasing likelihood that he or she will be placed in a foster or institutional setting. The flow of federal dollars heavily favors out-of-home care at the expense of preventive services that could maintain children in their own homes. We do not even know exactly how many children are in out-of-home care–there is a marked lack of reliable data despite clear data collection mandates. The figure is in the vicinity of half a million. Clearly, the removal of children from their homes without provision of family treatment is the most potentially harmful element of the present system.

Almost nothing has been done at the federal level to facilitate structural links among CPS, juvenile justice, mental health, schools, and other systems that deal with the older child. The lack of coordination often has horrendous consequences for children and their families. Without a mechanism for responding comprehensively to the needs of the child and the family, children are falling through the cracks as they pass from one single problem system to another. Families who need services face a maze of unresponsive agencies, each of whom views the child and family in terms of the services or training provided by that agency while ignoring other problems that are causing or contributing to the situation.

The traditional separation of CPS, juvenile justice, mental health, and school systems along categorical and departmental lines no longer makes sense. More communities are actively working to coordinate services across agencies, but efforts at the state and federal level have been minimal. We need to develop a cohesive approach to dysfunctional families based on an understanding of child development and family dynamics. Political disagreements over the desirability of certain goals and how those goals should be achieved must be resolved. Joint funding of programs and multisystem training are needed. Workers in all agencies must be able to assess both the troubled older child in the context of his or her family and the family in terms of its class, culture, and stressful life circumstances.

CONCLUSION

Prior to this study, research on the older maltreated child was minimal. Although numerous studies have reported that many dropouts, delinquents, runaways, suicide attempters, and teenage mothers had a history of abuse or neglect, these studies were unable to show that the maltreatment caused the problems. By documenting the severe consequences of maltreatment for school-age children (especially those who have been physically abused), this study takes us one step closer to establishing the causative links. Since our study began, the maltreated children who participated have dropped out of school in large numbers, committed delinquent acts, run away, been committed to a mental hospital for suicidal behavior, become pregnant, and given birth. None of the comparison group children had experienced such life disruptions by follow-up.

This chapter has suggested that troubled children and families are entering the child welfare system by a variety of routes–CPS, juvenile justice, mental health, runaway centers, etc.–but there is every indication that these children and families are interchangeable. If they are lucky, they find their way into the most benign system in their jurisdiction or live in a progressive community with updated practices and an array of quality services. But many are not so lucky. The resource limitations reported in this chapter are the rule, not the exception.

It is crucial that we acknowledge current system flaws and advocate essential improvements. Without people of vision leading the way, we will continue spending large amounts of money on out-of-home care that would be better spent on upgrading staff and providing services that could keep children in their homes and help families resolve their problems. Budgetary restrictions are not likely to let up in the foreseeable future, but rest assured, there is much that can be done. The next chapter will discuss a variety of approaches to serving the maltreated-multiproblem older child. We will recommend specific changes in policy, practice, and consciousness that should be implemented at all levels within and across systems.

NOTES

1. U.S. Advisory Board on Child Abuse and Neglect, *Child Abuse and Neglect: Critical First Steps in Response to a National Emergency* (Washington, DC: U.S. Government Printing Office, 1990).

2. Children's Defense Fund, *A Children's Defense Budget: An Analysis of the President's FY 1984 Budget and Children* (Washington, DC: Children's Defense Fund, 1983).

3. B.J. Meddin and I. Hansen, "The Services Provided During a Child Abuse and/or Neglect Case Investigation and the Barriers That Exist to Service Provision," *Child Abuse and Neglect* 9 (1985), 175-82.

4. J. Garbarino and S. McHale, "Introduction," *Children and Youth Services Review* 5 (1983): 5.

5. American Humane Association, *National Analysis of Official Child Neglect and Abuse Reporting. 1976* (Denver: American Humane Association, 1978).

6. D.J. Besharov, *Recognizing Child Abuse: A Guide for the Concerned* (New York: Free Press, 1990).

7. L. Brown, "Seeking a National Consensus," *Public Welfare* (Winter 1987): 12-17.

8. Select Committee on Children, Youth, and Families, *Abused Children in America: Victims of Official Neglect* (Washington, DC: U.S. Government Printing Office, 1987).

9. J. Hansen, *Suffer the Children* (Atlanta: Atlanta Journal-Constitution, special reprint of articles published June 4-10 1989).

10. Select Committee on Children, Youth, and Families, *Abused Children.*

11. J.T. Pardeck, "Multiple Placement of Children in Foster Family Care: An Empirical Analysis," *Social Work* 29 (1984): 506-9.

12. Select Committee on Children, Youth, and Families, *Abused Children.*

13. Select Committee on Children, Youth, and Families, *No Place to Call Home: Discarded Children in America* (Washington, DC: U.S. Government Printing Office, 1989).

14. Ibid.

15. J. Hansen, *Suffer the Children.*

16. D. Fanshel and E.B. Shinn, *Children in Foster Care: A Longitudinal Investigation* (New York: Columbia University Press, 1978).

17. Select Committee on Children, Youth, and Families, *No Place to Call Home.*

18. M.B. Mushlin, L. Levitt, and L. Anderson, "Court-Ordered Foster Family Care Reform: A Case Study," *Child Welfare* 65 (1986): 141-54.

19. J. Hansen, *Suffer the Children.*

20. Select Committee on Children, Youth, and Families, *No Place to Call Home.*

21. G. Frank, "Treatment Needs of Children in Foster Care," *American Journal of Orthopsychiatry* 50 (1980): 256-63; M. Swire and F. Kavaler, "Health Supervision of Children in Foster Care," *Child Welfare* 57 (1978): 563-9.

22. Select Committee on Children, Youth, and Families, *No Place to Call Home.*

23. J. Hansen, *Suffer the Children.*

24. National Center on Child Abuse and Neglect, *Study Findings. Study of National Incidence and Prevalence of Child Abuse and Neglect: 1988* (Washington, DC: U.S. Government Printing Office, 1988).

25. C.J. Garbarino, C.J. Schellenbach, and I.M. Sebes, *Troubled Youth, Troubled Families* (New York: Aldine, 1986).

26. Select Committee on Children, Youth, and Families, *No Place to Call Home.*

27. H.A. Davidson, "The Revolution in Family Law: Confronting Child Abuse," in *Perspectives on Child Maltreatment in the Mid '80s,* ed. National Center on Child Abuse and Neglect (Washington, DC: National Center on Child Abuse and Neglect, 1984): 35-39.

28. J. Hansen, *Suffer the Children.*

29. M.E. Pate, "If We Don't Want Violence, Let's Do Something About Abuse," *Justice for Children* 1 (1986): 16-17.

30. C.P. Smith, T.E. Black, and F.R. Campbell, *A National Assessment of Case Disposition and Classification in the Juvenile Justice System: Inconsistent Labeling,* vol. 1, *Process Description and Summary* (Washington, DC: Office of Juvenile Justice and Delinquency Prevention, 1980).

31. E. Farber, "The Maltreated Adolescent: Patterns of Physical Abuse," *Child Abuse and Neglect* 9 (1985): 201-6; M. Saltonstall, *Bridge Over Troubled Waters. Runaways and Youth on the Streets of Boston: One Agency's Response* (Boston: Boston Globe Foundation, 1984).

32. Select Committee on Children, Youth, and Families, *Youth and the Justice System: Can We Intervene Earlier?* (Washington, DC: U.S. Government Printing Office, 1984).

33. R.H. Andrews and A.H. Cohn, "PINS Processing in New York: An Evaluation," in *Beyond Control: Status Offenders in the Juvenile Court,* ed. L. E. Teitelbaum and A. R. Gough (Cambridge: Ballinger, 1977): 45-114.

34. New York State Assembly Committee on Child Abuse, *Report on the Relationship Between Child Abuse and Neglect and Later Socially Deviant Behavior* (New York: New York State Assembly, 1978).

35. Select Committee on Children, Youth, and Families, *No Place to Call Home.*

36. P.T. Howing, J.S. Wodarski, J.M. Gaudin, Jr., and P.D. Kurtz, "Effective Interventions to Ameliorate the Incidence of Child Maltreatment: The Empirical Base," *Social Work* 34 (1989): 330-8; D. Daro, *Confronting Child Abuse: Research for Effective Program Design* (New York: Free Press, 1988).

37. Select Committee on Children, Youth, and Families, *No Place to Call Home.*

38. W.C. Morse, *The Education and Treatment of Socioemotionally Impaired Children and Youth* (Syracuse: Syracuse University Press, 1985).

39. C. Jencks, M. Smith, H. Acland, M.J. Bane, D. Cohen, H. Gintin, B. Heyns, and S. Michelson, *Inequality: A Reassessment of the Effect of Family and Schooling in America* (New York: Harper & Row, 1972).

40. M. Rutter, B. Maughan, P. Mortimore, and J. Ouston, *Fifteen Thousand Hours* (London: Open Books, 1979); M. Rutter, "School Effects on Pupil Progress: Research Findings and Policy Implications," *Child Development* 54 (1983): 1-29.

41. C.P. Smith, D.J. Berkman, and W.M. Fraser, *A Preliminary National Assessment of Child Abuse and Neglect and the Juvenile Justice System: The Shadows of Distress* (Washington, DC: U. S. Department of Justice, Office of Juvenile Justice and Delinquency Prevention, 1980).

Chapter Eight

What We Need To Do

Although this study was specifically concerned with the consequences of abuse and neglect on the school-age child's development, our findings lend themselves to much broader interpretation and recommendations. The severe developmental delays and family difficulties we found for older maltreated children call for systemic as well as individual remedies. It is apparent that child maltreatment is not a singular problem, especially when older children are involved. The swarm of troubles surrounding child abuse and neglect–stress, alcohol and drug abuse, marital conflict, parental depression, school failure, dropping out, delinquency, emotional disturbance, teen pregnancy and substance abuse, running away, suicide threats, etc.–are not easily separated into problems for CPS (Child Protective Services), juvenile justice, mental health, and school systems. Interventions that deliver isolated services for symptomatic behaviors ignore the deeper meaning of behaviors and do little to foster family stability. When systems concentrate only on the parents or the child, underlying family problems may remain hidden and inaccessible to treatment.

Fundamental structural and functional changes are necessary if we expect our child and family service system to become an effective change agent. The variety of agencies that serve maltreated children need to operate from a set of common goals focused on families rather than isolated problems of individual family members. We need to move away from theoretical frameworks that rely on a simplistic, linear view of causality in which parents or children are treated according to outdated ideas and practices rather than current knowledge of what is effective. Both parents and children can accept age-appropriate responsibility for their own behaviors more easily if they are not pitted against each other by shortsighted agency policies.

This chapter will present policy and practice guidelines for improving services to school-age maltreated children and their families. Each child-serving agency has a vital role to play in reform efforts.

CPS REFORMS

Our public child welfare system has been moving toward a family preservation stance since the 1970s, but the flow of dollars still favors family breakup. Too often, the first-line solution in a child maltreatment case is to remove the child from the home. Instead, as official guidelines advise, a spectrum of family-based services should be provided to families, such as:

- emergency financial assistance
- emergency housing
- family, group, marital, and individual counseling
- home visits
- parenting education
- parent aide or homemaker services
- 24-hour crisis intervention
- emergency respite care centers for older children
- transportation
- advocacy
- drug and alcohol counseling
- employment counseling

These services may sound expensive, but they are far less costly than foster care placement which, in any case, leaves the underlying family problems unresolved and siblings at risk. The evidence is growing that family-based services are both effective in preventing placement and cost-effective compared to placement.[1] The program components considered most effective on both counts include group and family counseling, parenting education, skill development classes (especially for adolescents), peer support groups, lay therapy, and respite care.[2] Success depends on small caseloads (a maximum of 25 families, but preferably closer to 10), skilled caseworkers and supervisors, an adequate array of community services, and good collaboration with other agencies.

Family-centered placement prevention programs are operating in numerous communities across the country, but the majority of CPS families do not happen to live in these communities. The kinds of services these programs offer should be provided on a consistent, nationwide basis. However, this is not likely to happen without strong federal leadership. Congress should strengthen and expand fiscal incentives to states to transfer foster care maintenance funds to placement prevention services. It should provide guidelines and start-up costs for establishing family preservation programs.[3] Staffing increases should be the top priority. Hiring, training, and salary standards should reflect the specialized tasks CPS professionals are required to manage. Intervention should reflect our knowledge of how maltreating families change when effective services are provided.

Our study highlights the importance of providing direct therapeutic and remedial services to older maltreated children themselves, not just to their parents. It is particularly important that the children's school performance, behavior, and attendance be monitored and remediated. Physically abused older children (and those undergoing severe family stress or multiple foster care placements) should be assessed and treated for socioemotional problems. Caseworkers need to be informed of the specific developmental delays found in older abused and neglected children, and they need specialized training in how to assess and manage these cases. Policies and practices designed for the families of younger children are not always suitable for cases involving school-age children, especially adolescents. CPS agencies need to revise screening and service standards to ensure that acting-out adolescents who have been maltreated are not simply referred to the juvenile justice system.

Although foster care placements are considered a "treatment," placement often increases the child's distress.[4] School-age children placed in foster care are likely to need therapeutic services to help them deal with problems stemming from the traumatic events that led to placement, the separation from parents, and adjustment to foster care.[5] The timely provision of individual, group, and/or family therapy may be instrumental to avoiding placement disruption. In our study, children who had experienced multiple placements were maladjusted, aggressive, and low in self-concept. We do not know whether these socioemotional problems led to or resulted from the multiple placements but, in either case, the need for special services is clear.

Specialized foster care, in which higher than normal payments are made for more therapeutic foster care settings, is essential for older children whose symptoms and behaviors are problematic.[6] Children entering foster care should be comprehensively evaluated to identify their special needs and to ensure appropriate placement and community services. Recruitment and training of specialized foster parents should emphasize therapeutic approaches for dealing with children's educational and socioemotional deficits. Corporal punishment should be strictly prohibited in all foster care settings. Frequent home visits by caseworkers (at least once every two weeks) and weekly visits between the child and the natural parents should be standard.[7] Telephone contact in lieu of actual home visits is unacceptable.

Over the past decade, the foster care population has been growing older, and now nearly half of all foster children are adolescents.[8] There has been a growing recognition of the vulnerability of youth who age out of foster care before attaining self-sufficiency skills. Under federal legislation developed in 1986, many states and agencies have made considerable progress toward developing programs to prepare foster care adolescents for independent living.[9] However, the newness of the initiative, the lack of specific federal guidelines for programs, and the foot-dragging reluctance of the Department of Health and Human Services to support the initiative have hindered its implementation.[10] In many states, existing laws, licensing restrictions, and insurance requirements create obstacles to developing the services and alternate living arrangements that are needed.[11] A top priority is the delineation of nationwide standards for independent living services and guidelines for amending state laws to facilitate these services.

All foster children who are approaching emancipation should be provided life skills training that covers such areas as career and education planning; money management; home management; health maintenance; legal rights and responsibilities; community resources; and interpersonal, problem-solving, and self-control skills.[12] To facilitate the gradual transition from foster care to independent living, a range of options should be available. These may include:

- life skills training programs, conferences, and workshops
- specialized foster care and group homes that focus on teaching life skills and fostering independence
- supervised apartment houses monitored by adults who live in separate units on the premises
- apartment settings with live-in adult roommates who are trained to provide guidance
- boarding houses or host homes with adults who provide observation more than supervision
- supervised apartments that are monitored on a daily or weekly basis
- drop-in centers to provide supplemental services to former foster youth living on their own
- trained volunteers to serve as role models and mentors[13]

To provide a range of placement prevention and independent living services, CPS agencies can structure their operations in a number of ways. Services can be provided entirely by the agency itself or in conjunction with collateral public agencies. Or, as is increasingly the case, state and local CPS agencies can opt to purchase services from nongovernment organizations such as United Way agencies; voluntary child welfare organizations; nonprofit emergency shelters; private, for-profit counseling services; etc.[14] These organizations employ professional staff (and, often, volunteers) to provide either blanket services for maltreating families or specific service components such as counseling, skills training, homemaker assistance, respite care, or transportation services. Formal contracts specify the terms of service delivery, client eligibility, time limits, monitoring procedures, information exchange, fees, and payment procedures.

In many cases, contracting for nonpublic services may be more practical and cost-effective than providing the same services in-house.[15] The public sector's high administrative overhead; lack of sufficient staff, facilities, and specialized skills; and rigid civil service regulations make it difficult to establish new programs without a major infusion of new funds for start-up costs. Private agencies, on the other hand, usually have fewer bureaucratic constraints and more specialized expertise, rely more on volunteers, and are often able to augment contracted fees with donations. Purchase-of-services arrangements can increase the variety and availability of services, and the use of a bidding process for awarding contracts can encourage innovation and increase public control and accountability.[16]

Nevertheless, contracting for nonpublic services is hardly a cure-all for the CPS funding predicament. As with all new approaches, problems are surfacing that have yet to be resolved. When treatment components are subcontracted, roles, responsibilities, and treatment goals may become confused or conflicting.[17] The nonpublic sector may refuse to accept the neediest or most troublesome clients, and volunteers (who tend to be middle class and white) may be reluctant to make home visits to poor or minority neighborhoods.[18] Additionally, program effectiveness may be more difficult to assess when diverse services are provided under different auspices. Nonpublic agencies tend to resist close monitoring and may rely on inadequate methods of self-evaluation.[19]

As public agencies increasingly rely on purchasing services, they will have to increase their capacity to control, monitor, and evaluate the performance of outside service providers. Roles, responsibilities, and goals must be clearly defined prior to the implementation of services, and a mediation mechanism should be established early on to resolve disputes. Contracts should clarify which client characteristics are legitimate grounds for refusal to serve. In some cases, no-refusal contracts can be negotiated, or fiscal incentives can be offered for serving certain clients.[20] Service effectiveness should be evaluated through multicriteria outcome measures, including placement prevention, improvements in child and family functioning, and cost-effectiveness.

Whether services are purchased or CPS-based, they ought to reflect our current and evolving knowledge of maltreating families. The professional environment should include up-to-date literature and inservice training sessions that highlight important research findings. In a time of rapidly evolving knowledge, agencies must ensure that workers are apprised of current developments in the field and that they are supported when implementing research-based innovations.

JUVENILE JUSTICE SYSTEM REFORMS

The juvenile justice system frequently comes into contact with older maltreated children, and it has tremendous power to alter their life circumstances for good or ill. Far too often, this power is misapplied because severe staff and resource limitations allow for little more than the perfunctory processing of cases. Deep reforms are needed to assure that each case receives timely and thorough attention. As a starting point, all judges who handle child maltreatment cases should receive special training in the practical and developmental aspects of these cases. The American Bar Association's National Resource Center for Child Advocacy and Protection has developed training programs for this purpose.[21] It is essential that those individuals who have been appointed to serve on the juvenile court bench have a deep and knowledgeable commitment to the welfare of children.

Equally important, all abused or neglected children involved in judicial proceedings should be afforded independent representation (guardian ad litem) in accordance with federal law. Many communities are attempting to comply with the law by arranging for court-appointed lawyers, volunteer lawyers, law students, or trained volunteer lay persons to act as guardians ad litem. The most promising approach is the CASA (Court Appointed Special Advocate) Program, which has trained some 12,000 lay volunteers and served more than 67,000 children in 46 states.[22] CASA volunteers undergo extensive preservice and inservice training to prepare them for investigating cases, accompanying the child to court, and making recommendations to the judge. Research indicates that carefully selected and trained lay volunteers perform as well as lawyers and law students when representing maltreated children.[23]

Ultimately, if the courts are to play a meaningful role in addressing the problem of abuse and neglect, there must be substantial increases in staff and resources. To ensure that procedural safeguards are followed and treatment plans are carried out, court workers must have adequate time for case preparation, presentation, and monitoring. The courts should become more involved in the details of treatment planning and evaluation. They should not hesitate to use their power to help families by mandating participation in treatment programs when appropriate. Court-mandated treatment has proven effective in increasing parental involvement in treatment and improving parenting skills,[24] but success may depend on adequate court personnel for monitoring cases.

Some older maltreated children enter the juvenile justice system as recognized victims of abuse or neglect, but many others enter as offenders. Their equitable treatment requires a rethinking of current juvenile justice philosophy. Over the past few decades, a major policy shift has occurred in the field. The traditionally held rehabilitation model, which emphasized the needs of the youth over the seriousness of the offense, has given way to policy initiatives that undermine this principle. A new "get tough" movement has shifted the focus to punishing lawbreakers while "diverting" status offenders (acting-out youth).[25]

We have repeatedly argued that both delinquency and acting-out behaviors should be viewed as symptoms of underlying family problems. The juvenile justice system's current fixation on punishment, which is totally at odds with this view, is pervasive. Those youth who are not institutionalized receive few (if any) treatment services, and their parents are rarely involved in treatment. Government and foundation funding of research in juvenile justice is nowhere near the level afforded for child maltreatment research, and juvenile-justice-sponsored, family-based treatment programs are scarce. Because of large caseloads, juvenile probation officers typically provide minimal supervision and rely on threats of "consequences" to keep the youth in line.[26] Further, because violation of probation can bump a youth from status offender to delinquent, acting-out youth can end up in institutions intended for serious offenders.

A mass of evidence indicates that most juvenile offenders (both delinquent and status) experience some sort of family disturbance. In many cases, parental maltreatment clearly precipitates the deviant behavior. Abuse/neglect screening procedures should be required for every juvenile offender. Mechanisms need to be established for relabeling offenders as abused or neglected when maltreatment is recognized belatedly. When screening reveals family problems, a range of services should be offered or mandated, including counseling, family conflict mediation, parent education, respite care, family assistance, and specialized foster care. Serious maltreatment should be reported to CPS, as required by law, and services to the youth and family should be coordinated. Links between juvenile justice and CPS need to be fluid, with both systems focusing on the family in crisis rather than either the child or the parent.

There is no reason why CPS and juvenile justice clients could not make use of the same programs–the two populations surely form a continuum, with much overlapping of cases. Indeed, a few innovative juvenile justice programs reported in the literature sound much like the family-based intervention programs conducted under CPS auspices.[27] The joint funding of programs is especially plausible in light of the services purchasing trend sweeping the public sector. The juvenile justice system is no stranger to this trend: recently, the Office of Juvenile Justice and Delinquency Prevention funded a project (the Private Sector Probation Initiative) to study the feasibility of purchasing probation services from the private sector.[28] (We hope the services focus on families.)

A discussion of the justice system's role in maltreatment cases would be incomplete without mention of a seldom used but potentially powerful phenomenon, namely, court-ordered system reform. A precedent was established by the case of *G. L. v. Zumwalt* in which a federal court ordered comprehensive improvements in the entire foster care system of Jackson County, Missouri (including Kansas City).[29] The consent decree set enforceable minimum standards for 14 different aspects of foster care services, including caseload size, family visitation, foster parent training, and medical and mental health care for children in placement. Recent class-action lawsuits in Massachusetts, New Mexico, Connecticut, and Alabama have also set the stage for CPS reforms. Such legislation by court decree is controversial, but it may offer the best hope for improving child welfare services in some states and communities. When administrators' pleas to the legislative and executive branches for increased funding are repeatedly ignored, court-ordered reform can provide a powerful tool for assuring adequate funding.

MENTAL HEALTH SYSTEM REFORMS

Community mental health centers should play a much larger role in providing therapeutic services to maltreated children and their families. Currently, only the most seriously disturbed children receive services, and funds are inordinantly consumed by expensive residential placements. There needs to be a greater emphasis on early intervention, outpatient services, and family-based treatment. Jane Knitzer's *Unclaimed Children,* (1982) set the agenda for reform of children's mental health services.[30] Her recommendations, which would particularly benefit older maltreated children, include:

- creating a continuum of community-based services for troubled children and adolescents, with families involved in treatment as much as possible
- ensuring that children and adolescents receive a fair share of mental health funds
- establishing administrative child and adolescent units within state mental health departments
- providing increased training for mental health workers who counsel or make decisions regarding troubled children and adolescents
- extending Medicaid coverage of nonresidential mental health services to children and adolescents

Since Knitzer's study was published, targeted funds for outpatient child and adolescent services were resurrected through the federal Child and Adolescent Service System Program (CASSP). (Funding levels, however, are far lower than they should be.)

For the older maltreated child, the continuum of community mental health services should emphasize individual, group, and family counseling; peer support groups; and life skills training. Many maltreated children will welcome and take advantage of such therapeutic services; others will resist treatment, or their parents will not transport them to sessions on a regular basis. To overcome these obstructions, there must be strong links between mental health and CPS. In certain cases, court-ordered participation may be necessary, with parents held responsible for their child's attendance.

Community mental health centers need to become more involved with the issue of child abuse and neglect, and not just leave this problem up to CPS. Mental health practitioners should take part in outreach programs that foster awareness of the problem and of available community resources. Children and adolescents are frequently unaware of mental health resources and reluctant to seek professional help.[31] Outreach efforts can include dissemination of brochures, announcements on bulletin boards, articles in school newsletters, and speakers in class.[32] To increase utilization of mental health resources, services should accommodate the needs of youth through such means as:

- geographic accessibility
- late afternoon and evening hours
- drop-in times rather than appointments
- free services to those unable to pay
- ethnically and culturally diverse staff
- assurance of anonymity and confidentiality[33]

Mental health agencies are the most logical sponsors of comprehensive services for troubled families. Family-based intervention programs should be established under mental health auspices to serve all families with children at risk of placement, including CPS and juvenile justice clients. Programs such as Homebuilders (Tacoma, Washington), Intensive Family Services (Oregon), and Families, Inc. (West Branch, Iowa), report excellent results in keeping multiproblem families together.[34] The National Resource Center on Family Based Services (headquartered at the University of Iowa School of Social Work) conducts conferences, disseminates information on family-based programs, and publishes a quarterly newsletter.[35] Their efforts should be strongly supported.

EDUCATION REFORMS

During the past decade, and especially since the publication of *A Nation at Risk* in 1983, there has been a flurry of educational reform activity.[36] In Georgia, as in many states, the legislature has issued a barrage of new directives prescribing in great detail how children are to be taught and what they are expected to learn, with an emphasis on test scores.[37] Confronted with new performance demands and paperwork requirements, and lacking alternative resources and administrative support, teachers find less time to give individual attention to students' problems. What Brendtro and Mitchell call a "child-processing bureaucracy"[38] is emerging, and it cannot respond effectively to the special needs of older maltreated children and others who display academic and behavioral problems at school.

Reform efforts that impose rigid external standards may exact superficial compliance, but they do not produce effective schools (i.e., schools that are capable of fostering high achievement in all students). Studies have established that successful schools depend primarily on site-specific human factors: strong leadership; a high-quality instructional staff; and an orderly, supportive school climate.[39] The research shows that staff salary levels are more critical to student achievement than such factors as facilities and supplies, class and school size, number of administrators, tenure, or certification. Funding decisions should reflect these findings by ensuring that salary levels are high enough to attract and retain the best teachers and administrators. It is they who make the difference.

Research on effective schools particularly emphasizes the importance of the school principal in setting the tone for a positive school climate where staff morale and school spirit are high. The most effective principals create schools that are models of justice where staff and students (*all* students) are treated with genuine respect; where academic and discipline policies are clear and fair; and where administrators, teachers, students, and parents all participate in decision making and problem solving. No teacher should be expected to deal with severely disruptive students single-handedly or to spend excessive time on meaningless paperwork. No student should be subjected to corporal punishment or repeated out-of-school suspensions; no student should be summarily excluded from extracurricular activities for academic deficiencies; and no student should be failed because of behavior or absences. Certainly, the practice of promoting low-achieving students until they are old enough to drop out is unconscionable.

A positive school climate converts troubles into prime learning events, where problem solving is the lesson of the day–every day. Above all, schools need personnel who are skilled in conflict resolution strategies that keep the focus on here-and-now interactions, effective communication, empathy, clarification of distorted perceptions, and effective resolution rather than on blame and punishment. The goal is to resolve stressful situations so that long-term negative effects (e.g., alienation, failure, expulsion, dropping out–including dropping out by teachers!) are avoided and self-direction is enhanced. Schools can develop positive learning climates through inservice training,[40] school climate projects,[41] crisis intervention teachers or teams,[42] and/or the use of teacher consultants.[43] For older maltreated children, school-based interventions may provide their only exposure to effective problem-solving processes. Parents can also benefit from participation in these events, and they should be included when feasible.

Every effort should be made to enlist parents and other adults as participants in a positive school environment. These volunteers can serve as classroom resources and aides, advisors (e.g., through parent councils), and channels to the community. School policies should reflect the indisputable fact that families are crucial to children's academic achievement and, further, that parents and children today have many more problems than before. The schools (along with other agencies, churches, businesses, and volunteer organizations) must be asked to take an active role in ongoing and persistent outreach efforts. Administrators and teachers should be trained in techniques to involve parents. Once teachers understand that uninvolved or antagonistic parents are often defensive out of fear, shame, discomfort, suspicion, ethnic differences, stressed circumstances, and the like,[44] they may be more willing to help. As a starting point, the structure and timing of parent-teacher conferences should be modified to accommodate single parents and working parents, and contacts with parents should become less formal and "jargonized."[45] Another priority is establishing parent education programs within the schools (with fees waived for those who cannot afford to pay and special effort expended to involve parents of at-risk students).[46]

Teachers and administrators need specific training in the areas of child abuse and neglect, not only to increase the identification and reporting of victims but to increase sensitivity to these children's special needs. Slow-learning, withdrawn, or disruptive students may be perceived differently when the source and nature of their difficulties are understood. School staff may then be more likely to persist in reaching out to troubled children and to remain calm in the face of provocative behavior. Both preservice and inservice training in the management of maltreated children are especially important for high school staff because their students are more likely than younger children to be mainstreamed rather than provided with special education services.[47]

The Education for All Handicapped Children Act gives all educationally handicapped and emotionally disturbed children the right to a free and appropriate education at public expense. However, the Act fails to specify what services are to be provided and by whom. This is a local decision that is made according to the customs and laws of the locality and, occasionally, to court cases that attempt to clarify what "appropriate education" entails. Federal guidelines are needed to standardize the widely divergent special education practices that have evolved, and to prevent costly lawsuits. Guidelines are especially needed for services to older children and adolescents, who need more options than just mainstreaming or segregation into special classes.[48]

Clarification regarding the treatment of socioemotionally impaired (SEI) children (like the physically abused children we studied) is a particular priority. There is considerable confusion over which of these children are eligible for special education services under the Act, which specifically excludes "children who are socially maladjusted, unless it is determined that they are seriously emotionally disturbed."[49] The ruling has been interpreted and applied in markedly different ways, but the general absence of SEI programs in school districts across the country indicates that many school administrators have excluded antisocial and behavior-disordered students from special education mandates.[50] This practice "is not supported by research, scholarly opinion, or good professional practice,"[51] and undoubtedly contributes to high dropout and expulsion rates.

The point, however, is not that all of these students should be certified as special education students, but rather that social maladjustment should be recognized as a handicap that interferes with academic performance.[52] SEI students who are at risk of school failure or dropping out need appropriate services, with or without certification. Many school districts have established alternative education services for at-risk students who are not certified.[53] These include:

- alternative schools or classes
- in-school suspension programs featuring counseling and family treatment services
- vocational, work apprenticeship, and life skills programs
- special resource teams to provide intensive services
- independent study arrangements
- home-school liaison and parent assistance
- summer programs
- peer counseling
- outdoor challenge programs

Successful programs often feature: (1) small classes; (2) a non-traditional curriculum and/or environment; (3) committed teachers who are in the program by choice; (4) program autonomy; and (5) a flexible, individualized approach to students' academic and socioemotional needs.[54]

Specialized services often involve the larger community. Many schools have developed collaborative arrangements with outside organizations (e.g., businesses, universities, advisory committees) to provide instructors, tutors, equipment and materials, work-training programs, apprenticeships, scholarships and awards, internships, sites and funding for special programs, career counseling, placements for student teachers, and staff development activities.[55] Initiatives such as these can create schools with powerful economic and social inducements for troubled youth to stay in or return to school.

By the year 2000, the percentage of disadvantaged, at-risk, and educationally handicapped children coming into our school systems is likely to increase.[56] Piecemeal reforms that focus on narrow issues such as competence testing, school violence, vandalism, or drug abuse are not likely to produce schools that will be effective with these students. If older maltreated children and others with academic and socioemotional problems are to be adequately served by our school systems, the basic framework of education must be reformulated. The emphasis must be placed on staff quality, positive school climates, and change from within.

COORDINATION OF SERVICES

No single child-serving system has the solution to the problems of child abuse and neglect; older maltreated children and their families are likely to require many community resources. Federal guidelines have mandated increased communication, coordination, and joint planning among existing systems, but the increasing scope and decentralization of child and family services impede state and local efforts in this direction. Ultimately, the structural and functional division of CPS, juvenile justice, mental health, schools, and other child-serving systems should be questioned. To eliminate service gaps and minimize service duplication, we need a unified child and family service system in which boundaries are permeable and treatment goals are in accord across subsystems. In the meantime, we must continue moving toward the coordination of existing services.

Coordination can occur in a variety of ways. Informal collaboration–where two organizations consult on a case without formal agreement, reimbursement, or transfer of control functions–is the simplest and most common form of service coordination. For example, a CPS worker might contact a child's teacher, counselor, or juvenile worker to discuss the child's treatment needs, resolve difficulties, or advocate on behalf of the child. In other cases, more formal agreements between two agencies occur, as, for example, when a special education student's Individualized Education Program (IEP) stipulates that mental health counseling will be provided through special education funds.

Such ad hoc collaborative arrangements between two agencies may or may not prove effective, depending on the ability of individual workers to communicate across system boundaries and transcend traditional problems of "turfism." To address these deep-seated problems and foster a consistent, effective community response to child maltreatment, a more comprehensive collaborative approach is necessary. Community child protection councils are needed at the state and local level to facilitate both communication and the coordination of services among the various agencies that become involved with maltreated children and their families. These councils should not limit their purview to children who are formally identified as maltreated, but should focus on coordinating services for all troubled children (many of whom may be suffering from undetected maltreatment).

Federal standards emphasize that such councils should focus on agency structure and policies, community needs assessments, program planning and development, and the formation of multidisciplinary case consultation teams.[57] Thus far, coordination efforts in communities across the country have focused largely on establishing case consultation teams to review individual cases in terms of case management and treatment planning.[58] Since most of these teams include representatives from CPS, mental health organizations, schools, and the court system (though not usually those court workers who are involved with delinquent or status offenders), cooperative interagency relationships are likely to be enhanced through the team process. However, when the focus is on the management of individual cases, larger system issues may not be specifically addressed. Case consultation teams are a step in the right direction, but certainly should not be viewed as the endpoint in coordination efforts.

Substantial improvements in multiagency service delivery to maltreated and troubled children will not occur until service gaps and barriers are identified and addressed through long-range planning and changes in legislation, policies, and funding mechanisms. Community child protection councils should focus on this level of coordination by working to (1) define minimal standards of service,

(2) develop models for community treatment services, (3) propose specific legislation, and (4) foster public awareness and involvement. Coordination and planning efforts should particularly address the problem of maltreated older children who come in contact with the juvenile justice system or who are at risk of school failure or dropping out.

One way to facilitate interagency coordination is to provide joint training for administrators and workers from different agencies.[59] Such training ought to focus on increasing the level of knowledge about, and sensitivity to, issues of child maltreatment and family dysfunction. A dynamic educational process is crucial to the development of common treatment goals and service orientations. The feasibility of jointly sponsored programs should also be explored. Though challenging to develop, such programs can offer striking benefits for troubled children and their families. For example, mental health mini-clinics located within schools "on the wrong side of the tracks" can provide family treatment services where they are most needed.[60] Such efforts must be adequately evaluated and the findings disseminated in order to expand and refine new approaches to collaboration and coordination.

CONCLUSION

This chapter has focused on what we need to do to ensure adequate assistance for older maltreated children and their families. The first step is to acknowledge that our child and family service system is in a state of crisis. We need to face the facts and declare that we, as a society, will not tolerate the human suffering and the long-term costs of current policies and practices.

Second, we must grapple with fundamental issues and clearly define our minimum expectations for parenting, state interventions, and education. We need to conduct a thorough assessment of the current system and set priorities for federal, state, and community reform efforts. The U.S. Advisory Board on Child Abuse and Neglect has begun this process with the publication of its first report, which recommends 31 "critical first steps" in restructuring our response to child maltreatment.[61]

Finally, we must work to develop a coordinated range of community-based services for children and families in crisis. A piecemeal approach will not be sufficient. Fundamental structural changes are needed. This means strong federal involvement is necessary to fund and guide an integrated system that is directed toward the comprehensive assistance of families in crisis.

Certainly, there are major obstacles to overcome when creating bona fide multisystem reform, but the issue cannot be deferred to other times. We have shown that the consequences of maltreatment are serious for school-age children, especially those who have been physically abused. The systems designed to help these children cannot do the job without policy leadership, increased funding, and clear guidelines for the cross-system coordination of child and family services. This agenda should be elevated to the highest priority by citizens and elected officials. Those with the capability to do so should begin now to implement reform measures in every way possible. They should make it clear to higher-ups–from supervisors and administrators to mayors, legislators, and the president–that more must be done. Implementing the needed services and reforms may be difficult and costly, but the cost of inaction will be far, far higher in the long run.

NOTES

1. K. Nelson, A. Emlen, M.J. Landsman, and J. Hutchinson, *Factors Contributing to Success and Failure in Family-Based Child Welfare Services* (Iowa City, IA: University of Iowa, National Resource Center on Family Based Services, 1988); P. AuClaire and I.M. Schwartz, *An Evaluation of the Effectiveness of Intensive Home-Based Services as an Alternative to Placement for Adolescents and Their Families* (Minneapolis, MN: University of Minnesota, Hubert H. Humphrey Institute of Public Affairs, 1986); Select Committee on Children, Youth, and Families, *Abused Children in America: Victims of Official Neglect* (Washington, DC: U.S. Government Printing Office, 1987); J.A. Rosenthal and G.V. Glass, "Comparative Impacts of Alternatives to Adolescent Placement," *Journal of Social Service Research* 13, no. 3 (1990), 19-37.

2. D. Daro, *Confronting Child Abuse: Research for Effective Program Design* (New York: Free Press, 1988); K. Subramanian, "Reducing Child Abuse Through Respite Center Intervention," *Child Welfare* 64, no. 5 (1985): 501-9.

3. Select Committee on Children, Youth, and Families, *No Place to Call Home: Discarded Children in America* (Washington, DC: U.S. Government Printing Office, 1989); U.S. Advisory Board on Child Abuse and Neglect, *Child Abuse and Neglect: Critical First Steps in Response to a National Emergency* (Washington, DC: U.S. Government Printing Office, 1990).

4. E. Gil and K. Bogart, "Foster Children Speak Out: A Study of Children's Perceptions of Foster Care," *Children Today* 11 (1982): 7-9.

5. R. Molin, "Treatment of Children in Foster Care: Issues of Collaboration," *Child Abuse and Neglect* 12 (1988): 241-50.

6. L. Klee and N. Halfon, "Mental Health Care for Foster Children in California," *Child Abuse and Neglect* 11 (1987): 63-74; L.H. Boyd, Jr. and L.L. Remy, "Is Foster-Parent Training Worthwhile?" *Social Service Review* 52 (1978): 275-96.

7. M.B. Mushlin, L. Levitt, and L. Anderson, "Court-Ordered Foster Family Care Reform: A Case Study," *Child Welfare* 65, no. 2 (1986): 141-54.

8. American Public Welfare Association, *Voluntary Cooperation Information System Report* (Washington, DC: APWA, 1985).

9. E.V. Mech, ed., special issue, *Child Welfare* 67, no. 6 (1988).

10. M. Allen, K. Bonner, and L. Greenan, "Federal Legislative Support for Independent Living," *Child Welfare* 67, no. 6 (1988): 515-27.

11. M. Hardin, "New Legal Options to Prepare Adolescents for Independent Living," *Child Welfare* 67, no. 6 (1988): 529-46.

12. T. Tatara, P.R. Casey, K.L. Nazar, F.K. Richmond, R. Diethorn, and T. Chapmond, "Evaluation of Independent-Living Programs," *Child Welfare* 67, no. 6 (1988): 609-23.

13. M.J. Kroner, "Living Arrangement Options for Young People Preparing for Independent Living," *Child Welfare* 67, no. 6 (1988): 547-61; R. Cook, "Trends and Needs in Programming for Independent Living," *Child Welfare* 67, no. 6 (1988): 497-514; E.V. Mech and E.L. Leonard, "Volunteers as Resources in Preparing Foster Adolescents for Self-Sufficiency," *Child Welfare* 67, no. 6 (1988): 595-607.

14. H.W. Demone, Jr. and M. Gibelman, *Services for Sale: Purchasing Health and Human Services* (New Brunswick, NJ: Rutgers University Press, 1989); S. R. Smith, "The Changing Politics of Child Welfare Services: New Roles for the Government and the Nonprofit Sectors," *Child Welfare* 68, no. 3 (1989): 289-99.

15. Demone, *Services for Sale*; D. Fisk, H. Kiesling, and T. Mueller, *Private Provision of Public Services: An Overview* (Washington, DC: Urban Institute, 1978).

16. P.M. Kettner and L.L. Martin, *Purchase of Service Contracting* (Newbury Park, CA: Sage, 1987).

17. K. Miller, E. Fein, G. Bishop, and C. Murray, "Public-Private Collaboration and Permanent Planning," *Social Casework: The Journal of Contemporary Social Work* 66 (1985): 237-41; A.P. Fine and S.H. Fine, "Interagency Cooperation for the Delivery of Human Services: A Marketing Perspective," in *Services for Sale*: 121-30.

18. I. Wolock, "Contracting as a People-Processing Mechanism in a Public Child-Welfare Agency," in *Services for Sale*: 200-13; S. R. Smith, "The Changing Politics of Child Welfare Services: New Roles for the Government and the Nonprofit Sectors," *Child Welfare* 68, no. 3 (1989): 289-99.

19. P. Terrell, "Purchasing Social Services,"in *Encyclopedia of Social Work,* 18th ed., ed. National Association of Social Workers (Silver Spring, MD: NASW, 1987): 434-42; A. F. Hart, "Contracting for Child Welfare Services in Massachusetts: Emerging Issues for Policy and Practice," *Social Work* 33, no. 6 (1988): 511-15.

20. Smith, "The Changing Politics of Child Welfare Services."

21. National Legal Resource Center on Child Advocacy and Protection, ABA, 1800 M Street, Suite 200, Washington, DC 20036.

22. The Court-Appointed Special Advocate Committee, National Council of Family and Juvenile Court Judges, Judicial College Building, University of Nevada, Reno, NV 89507.

23. D.N. Duquette and S.H. Ramsey, "Using Lay Volunteers to Represent Children in Child Protection Court Proceedings," *Child Abuse and Neglect* 10 (1986): 293-308; J. Poertner and A. Press, "Who Best Represents the Interests of the Child in Court?" *Child Welfare* 69, no. 6 (1990): 537-49.

24. A.M. Irueste-Montes and F. Montes, "Court-Ordered vs. Voluntary Treatment of Abusive and Neglectful Parents," *Child Abuse and Neglect* 12 (1988): 33-39; D.A. Wolfe, J. Aragona, K. Kaufman, and J. Sandler, "The Importance of Adjudication in the Treatment of Child Abusers: Some Preliminary Findings," *Child Abuse and Neglect* 4 (1980): 127-35.

25. E.F. McGarrell, *Juvenile Correctional Reform: Two Decades of Policy and Procedural Change* (Albany, NY: State University of New York Press, 1988).

26. I.M. Schwartz, *(In)Justice for Juveniles: Rethinking the Best Interests of the Child* (Lexington, MA: D.C. Heath and Company, 1989).

27. R.M. Kagan, W.M. Reid, S.E. Roberts, and J. Silverman-Pollow, "Engaging Families of Court-Mandated Youths in an Alternative to Institutional Placement," *Child Welfare* 66, no. 4 (1987): 365-76.

28. Office of Juvenile Justice and Delinquency Prevention, "Privatizing Juvenile Probation Services: Five Local Experiences," *NIJ Reports* (A Bimonthly Journal of the National Institute of Justice) 217 (November/December 1989): 10-12.

29. M.B. Mushlin, L. Levitt, and L. Anderson, "Court-Ordered Foster Family Care Reform: A Case Study," *Child Welfare* 65, no. 2 (1986): 141-54.

30. J. Knitzer, *Unclaimed Children: The Failure of Public Responsibility to Children and Adolescents in Need of Mental Health Services* (Washington, DC: Children's Defense Fund, 1982).

31. G.M. Christopher, P.D. Kurtz, and P.T. Howing, "Status of Mental Health Services for Youth in School and Community," *Children and Youth Services Review* 11 (1989): 159-74.

32. J.G. McCullagh, "Survival Strategies for School Social Workers," *Social Work in Education* 22 (1982): 5-15.

33. J.B. Jones, P.B. Numerow, and S. Philliber, "Adolescents' Use of a Hospital-Based Contraceptive Program," *Family Planning Perspectives* 14, no. 4 (1982): 224-31.

34. M.E. Bryce and J.C. Lloyd, eds., *Treating Families in the Home: An Alternative to Placement* (Springfield, IL: Charles C Thomas, 1980).

35. National Resource Center on Family Based Services, The University of Iowa School of Social Work, N240 Oakdale Hall, Iowa City, IA 52242.

36. National Commission on Excellence in Education, *A Nation at Risk: The Imperative for Educational Reform* (Washington, DC: U.S. Government Printing Office, 1983).

37. C.D. Glickman, "Has Sam and Samantha's Time Come At Last?" *Educational Leadership* 46, no. 8 (1989): 4-9.

38. L.K. Brendtro and M.L. Mitchell, "The Organizational Ethos: From Tension to Teamwork," in *Re-Educating Troubled Youth: Environments for Teaching and Treatment,* ed. L. K. Brendtro, A. E. Ness, and colleagues (Hawthorne, NY: Aldine, 1983): 93-106.

39. A.W. Block, *Effective Schools: A Summary of Research* (New York: Educational Research Service, 1983).

40. D. Lay and E. Duffner, "LSI Inservice Training Model for Regular Classroom Teachers," *Pointer* 25, no. 2 (1981): 54-60; T. Gordon, *Teacher Effectiveness Training* (New York: Weiden, 1974).

41. S.C. Purkey and M.S. Smith, "Effective Schools: A Review," *The Elementary School Journal* 83, no. 4 (1983): 427-52.

42. L.K. Brendtro and A.E. Ness, "The Life-Space Interview: A Re-examination," in *Re-educating Troubled Youth*: 177-201; P.A. Gallagher, *Teaching Students with Behavior Disorders: Techniques and Activities for Classroom Instruction,* 2nd ed. (Denver: Love, 1988): 271-92; R. Redl and D. Wineman, *Controls from Within* (New York: Free Press, 1952).

43. T.E. Heron and K.C. Harris, *The Educational Consultant: Helping Professionals, Parents, and Mainstreamed Students* (Rockleigh, NJ: Allyn and Bacon, 1982).

44. Fine, "Facilitating Home-School Relationships."

45. Ibid., 173.

46. M.J. Fine, *The Second Handbook on Parent Education: Contemporary Perspectives* (San Diego, CA: Academic Press, 1989).

47. W.C. Morse, *The Education and Treatment of Socioemotionally Impaired Children and Youth* (Syracuse: Syracuse University Press, 1985): 305-9.

48. Ibid.

49. U.S. Department of Health, Education, and Welfare, Office of Education, "Education of Handicapped Children: Implementation of Part B of the Education of the Handicapped Act" *Federal Register,* vol. 42, no. 163, (August 23, 1977): 42478.

50. D.M. Nelson and R.B. Rutherford, Jr., "Troubled Youth in the Public Schools" in *Understanding Troubled and Troubling Youth,* ed. P. E. Leone (Newbury Park, CA: Sage, 1990): 38-60.

51. Ibid., 40.

52. J.M. Kauffman, *Characteristics of Behavior Disorders of Children and Youth,* 4th ed. (Columbus, OH: Merrill, 1989).

53. S.E. Wells, *At-Risk Youth: Identification, Programs, and Recommendations* (Englewood, CO: Teacher Ideas Press, 1990); R.F. Kronick and C.H. Hargis, *Dropouts: Who Drops Out and Why–And the Recommended Action* (Springfield, IL: Charles C Thomas, 1990): 91-110; D. Safer, ed., *School Programs for Disruptive Adolescents* (Baltimore: University Park, 1982); W. Hathaway, C. Sheldon, and P. McNamara, "The Solution Lies in Programs That Work," in *Youth at Risk: A Resource for Counselors, Teachers, and Parents,* ed. D. Capuzzi and D.R. Gross (Alexandria, VA: American Association for Counseling and Development, 1989): 367-394; H.R. Reinert and A. Huang, *Children in Conflict: Educational Strategies for the Emotionally Disturbed and Behaviorally Disordered,* 3rd. ed. (Columbus, OH: Merrill, 1987): 188-194; C. Franklin, J.S. McNeil, and R. Wright, Jr., "School Social Work Works: Findings from an Alternative School for Dropouts," *Social Work in Education, 12* (3, 1990): 177-194.

54. S.E. Wells, *At-Risk Youth,* 23.

55. B.L. Jones and R.W. Maloy, *Partnerships for Improving Schools* (New York: Greenwood Press, 1988).

56. H. Hodgkinson, *Drugs Demographics: The Future is Here Today,* Presentation at the Fourth Annual Conference on Drug-Free Schools and Communities, June, 1990 (Falls Church, VA).

57. J.L. Jenkins, R.A. MacDicken, and N.J. Ormsby, *A Community Approach: The Child Protection Coordinating Committee* (Washington, DC: U.S. Government Printing Office, 1979).

58. B.B. Kaminer, A.H. Crowe, and L. Budde-Giltner, "The Prevalence and Characteristics of Multidisciplinary Teams for Child Abuse and Neglect: A National Survey," in *The New Child Protection Team Handbook,* ed. D.C. Bross, R.D. Krugman, M.R. Lenherr, D.A. Rosenberg, and B.D. Schmitt (New York: Garland, 1988): 548-67.

59. Select Committee on Children, Youth, and Families, *No Place to Call Home: Discarded Children in America* (Washington, DC: U.S. Government Printing Office, 1989).

60. D.O. Blatt and D.A. Starr, "A Thriving Mini-Clinic in a School Setting," in *Family Counseling in School Settings,* ed. W.M. Walsh and N.J. Giblin (Springfield, IL: Charles C Thomas, 1988): 119-31.

61. U.S. Advisory Board on Child Abuse and Neglect, *Child Abuse and Neglect: Critical First Steps in Response to a National Emergency* (Washington, DC: U.S. Government Printing Office, 1990).

Appendix

TABLE A. Demographic Characteristics of Abusive, Neglectful, and Nonmaltreating Families

Characteristic	Abused	Neglected	Nonmaltreating	p
Race (N)	(22)	(47)	(70)	.04
White	55%	81%	63%	
Black	45%	19%	37%	
Gender (N)	(22)	(47)	(70)	.35
Male	41%	43%	54%	
Female	59%	57%	46%	
Age of child (N)	(22)	(47)	(70)	.36
Mean	12.48	12.44	11.93	
Income[a] (N)	(19)	(38)	(70)	.0001
Less than $10,000	58%	82%	26%	
10,000 - 20,000	32%	8%	16%	
More than 20,000	10%	11%	58%	
Parent education[a] (N)	(18)	(35)	(69)	.0001
Less than 12th grade	66%	75%	23%	
High school grad	22%	17%	25%	
Post high school	11%	9%	52%	

Parent occupation[a] (N)	(16)	(34)	(67)	.0001
Unskilled	25%	38%	15%	
Semi-skilled	69%	62%	47%	
Administrative	6%	0%	37%	
Dual/single parent[b] (N)	(21)	(41)	(70)	.04
Two parent	38%	63%	69%	
Single parent	62%	37%	31%	
Mother's age at birth of target child (N)	(18)	(35)	(67)	.001
Range	13-37	11-33	15-37	
Median	22	20	24	
Family size[b] (N)	(22)	(47)	(70)	.03
2 (parent/child)	14%	4%	3%	
3 or 4	32%	36%	54%	
5 or more	54%	60%	43%	
Mean	4.59	5.09	4.37	

[a]foster parent responses omitted. [b]for foster cases, characteristics of natural families are presented.

Notes. SES is not controlled. Probabilities reported are from appropriate statistical procedures (numerical data chi square and analysis of variance). Reprinted, by permission of *Social Work.*

TABLE B. Differences in the School Performance of Abused, Neglected, and Nonmaltreated Children

Criterion	Abused			Neglected			Nonmaltreated			p
	N	M	SD	N	M	SD	N	M	SD	
Overall	22	2.74*	.65	46	2.42*	.71	69	3.57	.77	.03
Language	14	44.43	26.14	37	28.97*	24.62	63	67.38	27.54	.005
Reading	16	206.69	37.05	32	188.03*	19.84	59	226.37	25.11	.005
Math	14	42.36*	21.41	37	28.46*	23.74	62	72.52	24.31	.001
Working below par	20	2.25*	.94	44	2.16*	.92	65	3.15	1.04	.03
Learning below par	20	2.10*	.97	43	2.24*	.73	65	3.40	1.00	.001
Grade repeats	22	.64*	.66	47	.72	.71	70	.32	.65	.005
Absences	16	10.00	8.00	37	21.35*	17.72	62	4.52	4.14	.001

*$p < .05$ (significantly different from nonmaltreatment group).

Notes. Results reflect differences at initial data collection. Language = IOWA Test of Basic Skills, Language Total (percentile rank); Reading = Georgia Criterion Reference Test (Total Scale Score, Reading); Math = IOWA Test of Basic Skills, Math Total (percentile rank). Probabilities given in p column are for ANCOVA with SES as the covariate. Reprinted by permission of *Social Work*.

TABLE C. Differences in the Socioemotional Development of Abused, Neglected, and Nonmaltreated Children

Dimension	Abused		Neglected		Nonmaltreated		p
	M	SD	M	SD	M	SD	
Problem behavior at home	55.23*	32.48	39.09	19.97	27.39	20.2	.0005
Problem behavior at school	40.87*	32.85	42.43[a]	33.90	20.47	28.65	.05
Self-concept	47.09*	14.07	57.09	15.06	58.77	13.44	.009
Aggression	17.05*	5.65	12.04	4.83	12.86	4.36	.0001
School adjustment	17.39*	10.20	12.74	7.55	7.61	7.64	.001
Home adjustment	5.07*	3.61	3.33*	2.79	2.12	2.03	.0002
Emotional adjustment	17.59*	7.77	12.78	6.78	12.06	6.75	.007
Peer relationships	4.00*	2.83	2.09	2.11	1.52	2.00	.0001
Delinquency	8.46*	9.65	2.24	3.86	0.78	1.86	.0001

[a]Teacher reported problem behaviors are not significant for neglected children when both SES and race are controlled.

*$p < .05$ (significantly different from nonmaltreatment group by T-test).

Notes. N = 22 Abused, 47 Neglected, 70 Nonmaltreated. Results reflect differences at initial data collection. Problem behaviors = Child Behavior Checklist; self-concept = Piers-Harris Children's Self-Concept Scale; aggression = Jesness Manifest Aggression Subscale. Probabilities given in p column are for ANCOVA with SES as covariate. Reprinted, by permission of *Social Work.*

TABLE D. Changes in Child Functioning Over Time for Abused, Neglected, and Nonmaltreated Children on Various Measures (Low SES Subjects Only)

Measure	Abused		Neglected		Maltreated	
	N	M	N	M	N	M
Overall school performance	12	-.18	33	+.13*	18	-.15
Problem behavior at home	13	+12.23*	33	+7.27	18	-1.54
Problem behavior at school	13	-9.51	33	-6.87	18	+3.20
Self-concept	15	+4.86	34	+3.05	18	+4.39
Aggression	15	+.30	35	-.74	18	-.94
School adjustment	5	+3.00	19	-.41	11	-2.36
Home adjustment	15	+1.07	36	+1.43	18	+.97

Emotional adjustment	15	+1.34	36	+2.36	18	+1.11
Peer relationships	15	+1.20	36	+.48	18	+.11
Delinquency	15	+.86	36	-.64	18	-.61
Motor skills	13	+1.92	32	+5.41	18	-.77
Personal care skills	13	-3.30	32	+1.03	18	+2.64
Community skills	13	-1.23	32	+1.40	18	-1.94

*change over time is significantly different ($p < .05$) between experimental (abused or neglected) and comparison group.

Notes. Change scores are from repeated measures ANOVA. Direction of scoring was reversed in certain cases such that all positive change scores reflect improvement and all negative change scores reflect decline. Missing data accounts for variation in Ns. Problem Behaviors = Child Behavior Checklist; self-concept = Piers-Harris Children's Self-Concept Scale; aggression = Jesness Manifest Aggression Subscale; motor skills, personal care skills, community skills = Woodcock-Johnson Scales of Independent Behavior.

TABLE E. Mean Differences Between Maltreatment and Nonmaltreatment Families on Mediating and Control Variables

Mediating Variable	Abuse		Neglect		Nonmaltreated	
	N	M	N	M	N	M
Stress						
Stressful events	19	348.84*	38	377.42*	70**	207.07
Unemployment	17	.47	27	.51	59	.19
Single parent	16	.45	37	.44	70	.31
Marital conflict	19	1.00	38	1.08**	70	.50
Number of siblings	17	1.89	37	2.28	67	1.63
Social support	16	19.00	28	16.97	50	21.58
Parental depression	19	10.74**	38	9.11	70	8.01
Control Variables						
Parental aggression (self-reported)	19	1.07	38	1.18	70	.64
Child neglect (interviewer rating)	19	80.02**	36	62.96***	66	95.04

*p < .05
**p < .01
***p < .001

Notes. Probabilities given are for T-test differences from comparison group within ANCOVAs with SES as the covariate. Results reflect differences at initial data collection. With the exception of child neglect, higher scores indicate more negative functioning. Stressful life events = Life Events Inventory; parental aggression = Conflict Tactics Scale (physical aggression by self portion); child neglect = Child Well-Being Scales (three items).

Sources Cited

Aber, J.L., and D. Cicchetti. "The Socio-emotional Development of Maltreated Children." In *Theory and Research on Behavioral Pediatrics,* ed. B.M. Lester and M.W. Yogman, 147-205. New York: Plenum Press, 1984.

Achenbach, T.M., and C.S. Edelbrock. *Child Behavior Checklist.* Burlington, VT: University of Vermont, Center for Children, Youth, and Families, 1980.

Alfaro, J.D. "Report on the Relationship between Child Abuse and Neglect and Later Socially Deviant Behavior." In *Exploring the Relationship between Child Abuse and Delinquency,* ed. R.J. Hanner and Y.E. Walker, 175-219. Montclair, NJ: Allanheld, Osmun, and Company, 1981.

Allen, M., K. Bonner, and L. Greenan. "Federal Legislative Support for Independent Living." *Child Welfare* 67, no. 6 (1988): 515-527.

Ambrose, S., A. Hazzard, and J. Haworth. "Cognitive Behavioral Parenting Groups for Abusive Families." *Child Abuse and Neglect* 4 (1980): 119-124.

American Humane Association. *National Analysis of Official Child Neglect and Abuse Reporting 1976.* Denver: American Humane Association, 1978.

American Public Welfare Association. *Voluntary Cooperation Information System Report.* Washington, DC: APWA, 1985.

Andrews, R.H., and A.H. Cohn. "PINS Processing in New York: An Evaluation." In *Beyond Control: Status Offenders in the Juvenile Court,* ed. L.E. Teitelbaum and A.R. Gough, 45-114. Cambridge: Ballinger, 1977.

Barahal, R.M., J. Waterman, and H.P. Martin. "The Social Cognitive Development of Abused Children." *Journal of Consulting and Clinical Psychology* 49 (1981): 508-516.

Baumrind, D. "Authoritarian vs. Authoritative Parental Control." *Adolescence* 3 (1968): 255-272.

______. "Current Patterns of Parental Authority." *Developmental Psychology Monographs* 4 (1971): 99-103.

Belle, D., ed. *Lives in Stress: Women and Depression.* Beverly Hills: Sage, 1982.

Berger, K.S. *The Developing Person Through Childhood and Adolescence.* 2d ed. New York: Worth, 1986.

Besharov, D.J. *Recognizing Child Abuse: A Guide for the Concerned.* New York: Free Press, 1990.

Blatt, D.O., and D.A. Starr. "A Thriving Mini-Clinic in a School Setting." In *Family Counseling and School Settings,* ed. W.M. Walsh and N.J. Giblin, 119-31. Springfield, IL: Charles C Thomas, 1988.

Block, A.W. *Effective Schools: A Summary of Research.* New York: Educational Research Service, 1983.

Bousha, D.M., and C.T. Twentyman. "Mother-Child Interactional Style in Abuse, Neglect, and Control Groups: Naturalistic Observations in the Home." *Journal of Abnormal Psychology* 93 (1984): 106-114.

Boyd, L.H., Jr., and L.L. Remy. "Is Foster-Parent Training Worthwhile?" *Social Service Review* 52 (1978): 275-296.

Brendtro, L.K., and A.E. Ness. "The Life-Space Interview: A Reexamination." In *Re-educating Troubled Youth,* ed. L.K. Bendtro, A.E. Ness, and colleagues, 177-201. Hawthorne, NY: Aldine, 1983.

Brendtro, L.K., and M.L. Mitchell. "The Organizational Ethos: From Tension to Teamwork." In *Re-educating Troubled Youth: Environments for Teaching and Treatment,* ed. L.K. Bendtro, A.E. Ness, and colleagues, 93-106. Hawthorne, NY: Aldine, 1983.

Brown, L. "Seeking a National Consensus." *Public Welfare* (Winter 1987): 12-17.

Brown, S.E. "Social Class, Child Maltreatment, and Delinquent Behavior." *Criminology* 22 (1984): 259-278.

Browne, A., and D. Finkelhor. "Impact of Child Sexual Abuse: A Review of the Research." *Psychological Bulletin* 99 (1986): 66-77.

Bruininks, R.H., R.W. Woodcock, R.F. Weatherman, and B.K. Hill. *Scales of Independent Behavior: Woodcock-Johnson Psycho-*

educational Battery, Part IV. Allen, TX: DLM Teacher Resources, 1984.

Bryce, M.E., and J.C. Lloyd, eds. *Treating Families in the Home: An Alternative to Placement.* Springfield, IL: Charles C Thomas, 1980.

Burgess, R.L., and R.D. Conger. "Family Interaction Patterns Related to Child Abuse and Neglect: Some Preliminary Findings." *Child Abuse and Neglect* 1 (1977): 269-277.

Carnegie Corporation. *Turning Points: Preparing American Youth for the 21st Century.* New York: Carnegie Corporation, 1989.

Children's Defense Fund. *A Children's Defense Budget: An Analysis of the President's FY 1984 Budget and Children.* Washington, DC: Children's Defense Fund, 1983.

Christopher, G.M., P.D. Kurtz, and P.T. Howing. "Status of Mental Health Services for Youth in School and Community." *Children and Youth Services Review* 11 (1989): 159-174.

Cochrane, R., and A. Robertson. "The Life Events Inventory: A Measure of the Relative Severity of Psycho-social Stressors." *Journal of Psychosomatic Research* 17 (1973): 135-139.

Compas, B.E. "Stress and Life Events During Childhood and Adolescence." *Clinical Psychology Review* 7 (1987): 275-302.

Cook, R. "Trends and Needs in Programming for Independent Living." *Child Welfare* 67, no. 6 (1988): 497-514.

Coopersmith, S. *The Antecedents of Self-Esteem.* San Francisco: Freeman, 1967.

Dale, P., T. Morrison, M. Davies, P. Noyes, and W. Roberts. "A Family-Therapy Approach to Child Abuse: Countering Resistance." *Journal of Family Therapy* 5 (1983): 117-143.

Daro, D. *Confronting Child Abuse: Research for Effective Program Design.* New York: Free Press, 1988.

Davidson, H.A. "The Revolution in Family Law: Confronting Child Abuse." In *Perspectives on Child Maltreatment in the Mid '80s,* ed. National Center on Child Abuse and Neglect, 35-39. Washington, DC: National Center on Child Abuse and Neglect, 1984.

Demone, H.W., Jr., and M. Gibelman. *Services for Sale: Purchasing Health and Human Services.* New Brunswick, NJ: Rutgers University Press, 1989.

Duquette, D.N., and S.H. Ramsey. "Using Lay Volunteers to Represent Children in Child Protection Court Proceedings." *Child Abuse and Neglect* 10 (1986): 293-308.

Egeland, B., A. Sroufe, and M. Erickson. "The Developmental Consequences of Different Patterns of Maltreatment." *Child Abuse and Neglect* 7 (1983): 459-469.

Elmer, E. *Fragile Families, Troubled Children: The Aftermath of Infant Trauma.* Pittsburgh: University of Pittsburgh Press, 1977.

Erickson, M.F., B. Egeland, and R. Pianta. "The Effects of Maltreatment on the Development of Young Children." In *Child Maltreatment: Theory and Research on the Causes and Consequences of Child Abuse and Neglect,* ed. D. Cicchetti and V. Carlson, 647-684. New York: Cambridge University Press, 1989.

Erikson, E.H. *Childhood and Society.* 2d ed. New York: W.W. Norton, 1963.

Euster, S.D., V.P. Ward, J.G. Varner, and G.L. Euster. "Life Skills Group for Adolescent Foster Children." *Child Welfare* 63, no. 1 (1984): 27-36.

Fanshel, D., and E.B. Shinn. *Children in Foster Care: A Longitudinal Investigation.* New York: Columbia University Press, 1978.

Farber, E. "The Maltreated Adolescent: Patterns of Physical Abuse." *Child Abuse and Neglect* 9 (1985): 201-206.

Fine, A.P., and S.H. Fine. "Interagency Cooperation for the Delivery of Human Services: A Marketing Perspective." In *Services for Sale: Purchasing Health and Human Services,* 121-130. New Brunswick, NJ: Rutgers University Press, 1989.

Fine, M.J. *The Second Handbook on Parent Education: Contemporary Perspectives.* San Diego, CA: Academic Press, 1989.

Fisk, D., H. Kiesling, and T. Mueller. *Private Provision of Public Services: An Overview.* Washington, DC: Urban Institute, 1978.

Frank, G. "Treatment Needs of Children in Foster Care." *American Journal of Orthopsychiatry* 50 (1980): 256-263.

Franklin, C., J.S. McNeil, and R. Wright, Jr. "School Social Work Works: Findings from an Alternative School for Dropouts." *Social Work in Education* 12 (3, 1990): 177-194.

Gallagher, P.A. *Teaching Students with Behavior Disorders: Techniques and Activities for Classroom Instruction.* 2d ed. Denver: Love, 1988.

Garbarino, J. "The Human Ecology of Maltreatment: A Conceptual Model for Research." *Journal of Marriage and the Family* 39 (1977): 721-736.

Garbarino, J., and S. McHale. "Introduction." *Children and Youth Services Review* 5 (1983): 5.

Garbarino, C.J., C.J. Schellenbach, and I.M. Sebes. *Troubled Youth, Troubled Families: Understanding Families At-Risk for Adolescent Maltreatment.* New York: de Gruyter, 1986.

George, C., and M. Main. "Social Interactions of Young Abused Children: Approach, Avoidance, and Aggression." *Child Development* 50 (1979): 306-338.

Gil, E., and K. Bogart. "Foster Children Speak Out: A Study of Children's Perceptions of Foster Care." *Children Today* 11 (1982): 7-9.

Giovanni, J.M., and A. Billingsley. "Child Neglect Among the Poor: A Study of Parental Adequacy in Families of Three Ethnic Groups." *Child Welfare* 49 (1970): 196-206.

Glickman, C.D. "Has Sam and Samantha's Time Come At Last?" *Educational Leadership* 46, no. 8 (1989): 4-9.

Gordon, T. *Teacher Effectiveness Training.* New York: Weiden, 1974.

Hansen, J. *Suffer the Children.* Atlanta: Atlanta Journal-Constitution, special reprint of articles published June 4-10, 1989.

Hardin, M. "New Legal Options to Prepare Adolescents for Independent Living." *Child Welfare* 67, no. 6 (1988): 529-546.

Hart, A.F. "Contracting for Child Welfare Services in Massachusetts: Emerging Issues for Policy and Practice." *Social Work* 33, no. 6 (1988): 511-515.

Hathaway, W., C. Sheldon, and P. McNamara. "The Solution Lies in Programs That Work." In *Youth at Risk: A Resource for Counselors, Teachers, and Parents,* ed. D. Capuzzi and D.R. Gross, 367-394. Alexandria, VA: American Association for Counseling and Development, 1989.

Heron, T.E., and K.C. Harris. *The Educational Consultant: Helping Professionals, Parents, and Mainstreamed Students.* Rockleigh, NJ: Allyn and Bacon, 1982.

Hodges, K. "Assessing Children with a Clinical Research Interview: The Child Assessment Schedule." *Advances in Behavioral Assessment of Children and Families* 3 (1987): 203-233.

Hodgkinson, H. *Drugs Demographics: The Future Is Here Today.* Presentation at the Fourth Annual Conference on Drug-Free Schools and Communities, June, 1990 (Falls Church, VA).

Hoffman, M.L. "Moral Development." In *Carmichael's Manual of Child Psychology* 2d ed., ed. P.H. Mussen, 261-359. New York: Wiley, 1970.

Hoffman-Plotkin, D., and C.T. Twentyman. "A Multimodal Assessment of Behavioral and Cognitive Deficits in Abused and Neglected Preschoolers." *Child Development* 55 (1984): 794-802.

Howing, P.T., J.S. Wodarski, J.M. Gaudin, Jr., and P.D. Kurtz. "Effective Interventions to Ameliorate the Incidence of Child Maltreatment: The Empirical Base." *Social Work* 34 (1989): 330-338.

Hughes, F.P., L.D. Noppe, and I.C. Noppe. *Child Development.* Los Angeles: West Publishing Company, 1988.

Irueste-Montes, A.M., and F. Montes. "Court-Ordered vs. Voluntary Treatment of Abusive and Neglectful Parents." *Child Abuse and Neglect* 12 (1988): 33-39.

Jencks, C., M. Smith, H. Acland, M.J. Bane, D. Cohen, H. Gintin, B. Heyns, and S. Michelson. *Inequality: A Reassessment of the Effect of Family and Schooling in America.* New York: Harper & Row, 1972.

Jenkins, J.L., R.A. MacDicken, and N.J. Ormsby. *A Community Approach: The Child Protection Coordinating Committee.* Washington, DC: U.S. Government Printing Office, 1979.

Jesness, C.F. *Manual: The Jesness Inventory.* Palo Alto, CA: Consulting Psychologists Press, 1983.

Jewell, D.K. *Confronting Child Abuse Through Recreation.* Springfield, IL: Charles C Thomas, 1989.

Jones, B.L., and R.W. Maloy. *Partnerships for Improving Schools.* New York: Greenwood Press, 1988.

Jones, J.B., P.B. Numerow, and S. Philliber. "Adolescents' Use of a Hospital-Based Contraceptive Program." *Family Planning Perspectives* 14, no. 4 (1982): 224-31.

Kagan, R.M., W.M. Reid, S.E. Roberts, and J. Silverman-Pollow. "Engaging Families of Court-Mandated Youths in an Alternative to Institutional Placement." *Child Welfare* 66, no. 4 (1987): 365-376.

Kaminer, B.B., A.H. Crowe, and L. Budde-Giltner. "The Prevalence and Characteristics of Multidisciplinary Teams for Child Abuse and Neglect: A National Survey." In *The New Child Protection Team Handbook,* ed. D.C. Bross, R.D. Krugman, M.R. Lenherr, D.A. Rosenberg, and B.D. Schmitt, 548-567. New York: Garland, 1988.

Kauffman, J.M. *Characteristics of Behavior Disorders of Children and Youth.* 4th ed. Columbus, OH: Merrill, 1989.

Kent, J.T. "A Follow-Up Study of Abused Children." *Journal of Pediatric Psychology* 1 (1976): 25-31.

Kettner, P.M., and L.L. Martin. *Purchase of Service Contracting.* Newbury Park, CA: Sage, 1987.

Klee, L., and N. Halfon. "Mental Health Care for Foster Children in California." *Child Abuse and Neglect* 11 (1987): 63-74.

Knitzer, J. *Unclaimed Children: The Failure of Public Responsibility to Children and Adolescents in Need of Mental Health Services.* Washington, DC: Children's Defense Fund, 1982.

Koverola, C., D. Elliott-Faust, and D. Wolfe. "Clinical Issues in the Behavioral Treatment of a Child Abusive Mother Experiencing Multiple Life Stresses." *Journal of Clinical Child Psychology* 13 (1984): 187-191.

Kroner, M.J. "Living Arrangement Options for Young People Preparing for Independent Living." *Child Welfare* 67, no. 6 (1988): 547-561.

Kronick, R.F., and C.H. Hargis. *Dropouts: Who Drops Out and Why–And the Recommended Action.* Springfield, IL: Charles C Thomas, 1990.

Lahey, B.B., R.D.Conger, B.M. Atkinson, and F.A. Treiber. "Parenting Behavior and Emotional Status of Physically Abusive Mothers." *Journal of Consulting and Clinical Psychology* 52 (1984): 1062-1071.

Lay, D., and E. Duffner. "LSI Inservice Training Model for Regular Classroom Teachers." *Pointer* 25, no. 2 (1981): 54-60.

Lynch, M.A., and J. Roberts. *Consequences of Child Abuse.* London: Academic Press, 1982.

Maccoby, E.E. "Middle Childhood in the Context of the Family."

In *Development During Middle Childhood: The Years from Six to Twelve,* ed. W.A. Collins, 185-239. Washington, DC: National Academy Press, 1984.

Magura, S., and B.S. Moses. *Outcome Measures for Child Welfare Services: Theory and Application.* Washington, DC: Child Welfare League of America, 1986.

McCullagh, J.G. "Survival Strategies for School Social Workers." *Social Work in Education* 22 (1982): 5-15.

McGarrell, E.F. *Juvenile Correctional Reform: Two Decades of Policy and Procedural Change.* Albany, NY: State University of New York Press, 1988.

Mech, E.V., ed. Special issue, *Child Welfare* 67, no. 6 (1988).

Mech, E.V., and E.L. Leonard. "Volunteers as Resources in Preparing Foster Adolescents for Self-Sufficiency." *Child Welfare* 67, no. 6 (1988): 595-607.

Meddin, B.J., and I. Hansen. "The Services Provided During a Child Abuse and/or Neglect Case Investigation and the Barriers That Exist to Service Provision." *Child Abuse and Neglect* 9 (1985): 175-182.

Miller, K., E. Fein, G. Bishop, and C. Murray. "Public-Private Collaboration and Permanent Planning." *Social Casework: The Journal of Contemporary Social Work* 66 (1985): 237-241.

Molin, R. "Treatment of Children in Foster Care: Issues of Collaboration." *Child Abuse and Neglect* 12 (1988): 241-250.

Morris, M., and R. Gould. *The Neglected Battered Child Syndrome.* New York: Child Welfare League of America, 1975.

Morse, W.C. *The Education and Treatment of Socioemotionally Impaired Children and Youth.* Syracuse: Syracuse University Press, 1985.

Mouzakitis, C.M., and R. Varghese, eds. *Social Work Treatment with Abused and Neglected Children.* Springfield, IL: Charles C Thomas, 1988.

Mushlin, M.B., L. Levitt, and L. Anderson. "Court-Ordered Foster Family Care Reform: A Case Study." *Child Welfare* 65, no. 2 (1986): 141-154.

National Center on Child Abuse and Neglect. *Study Findings. Study of National Incidence and Prevalence of Child Abuse and Ne-*

glect: 1988. Washington, DC: U.S. Government Printing Office, 1988.

National Commission on Excellence in Education. *A Nation at Risk: The Imperative for Educational Reform.* Washington, DC: U.S. Government Printing Office, 1983.

Nelson, D.M., and R.B. Rutherford, Jr. "Troubled Youth in the Public Schools." In *Understanding Troubled and Troubling Youth,* ed. P.E. Leone, 38-60. Newbury Park, CA: Sage, 1990.

Nelson, K., A. Emlen, M.J. Landsman, and J. Hutchinson. *Factors Contributing to Success and Failure in Family Based Child Welfare Services.* Iowa City, IA: Univeristy of Iowa, National Resource Center on Family Based Services, 1988.

New York State Assembly Committee on Child Abuse. *Report on the Relationship Between Child Abuse and Neglect and Later Socially Deviant Behavior.* New York: New York State Assembly, 1978.

Office of Juvenile Justice and Delinquency Prevention. "Privatizing Juvenile Probation Services: Five Local Experiences." *NIJ Reports* (A Bimonthly Journal of the National Institute of Justice) 217 (November/December 1989): 10-12.

Pardeck, J.T. "Multiple Placement of Children in Foster Family Care: An Empirical Analysis." *Social Work* 29 (1984): 506-509.

Pate, M.E. "If We Don't Want Violence, Let's Do Something About Abuse." *Justice for Children* 1 (1986): 16-17.

Patterson, G.R. *A Social Learning Approach.* Vol. 3, *Coercive Family Process.* Eugene, OR: Castalia, 1982.

Piers, E.V. *Piers-Harris Children's Self-Concept Scale: Revised Manual 1984.* Los Angeles: Western Psychological Services, 1986.

Poertner, J., and A. Press. "Who Best Represents the Interests of the Child in Court?" *Child Welfare* 69, no. 6 (1990): 537-549.

Polanski, N.A., M.A. Chalmers, C. Buttenweiser, and D.P. Williams. "Isolation of the Neglectful Family." *American Journal of Orthopsychiatry* 49 (1979): 149-152.

Polanski, N.A., C. Hally, and N.F. Polanski. *Profile of Neglect–A Survey of the State of the Knowledge of Child Neglect.* Washington, DC: U.S. Department of Education and Welfare, Community Services Administration, 1975.

Purkey, S.C., and M.S. Smith. "Effective Schools: A Review." *The Elementary School Journal* 83, no. 4 (1983): 427-452.

Redl, R., and D. Wineman. *Controls from Within.* New York: Free Press, 1952.

Reinert, H.R., and A. Huang. *Children in Conflict: Educational Strategies for the Emotionally Disturbed and Behaviorally Disordered.* 3d ed. Columbus, OH: Merrill, 1987.

Richman, N. "Depression in Mothers of Preschool Children." *Journal of Child Psychology and Psychiatry* 17 (1976): 75-78.

Robins, L.N. "Sturdy Childhood Predictors of Adult Antisocial Behavior: Replications from Longitudinal Studies." *Psychological Medicine* 8 (1978): 611-622.

Rosenthal, J.A., and G.V. Glass. Comparative Impacts of Alternatives to Adolescent Placement." *Journal of Social Service Research* 13, no. 3 (1990): 19-37.

Rutter, M. "School Effects on Pupil Progress: Research Findings and Policy Implications." *Child Development* 54 (1983): 1-29.

Rutter, M., B. Maughan, P. Mortimore, and J. Ouston. *Fifteen Thousand Hours.* London: Open Books, 1979.

Safer, D., ed. *School Programs for Disruptive Adolescents.* Baltimore: University Park, 1982.

Saltonstall, M. *Bridge Over Troubled Waters. Runaways and Youth on the Streets of Boston: One Agency's Response.* Boston: Boston Globe Foundation, 1984.

Schaefer, C.F., and K.J. O'Connor, eds. *Handbook of Play Therapy.* New York: John Wiley, 1983.

Schwartz, I.M. *(In)Justice for Juveniles: Rethinking the Best Interests of the Child.* Lexington, MA: D.C. Heath and Company, 1989.

Schwartz, I.M., and P. AuClaire. *An Evaluation of the Effectiveness of Intensive Home-Based Services as an Alternative to Placement for Adolescents and Their Families.* Minneapolis, MN: University of Minnesota, Hubert H. Humphrey Institute of Public Affairs, 1986.

Seagull, E.A.W. "Social Support and Child Maltreatment: A Review of the Evidence." *Child Abuse and Neglect* 11 (1987): 41-52.

Select Committee on Children, Youth, and Families. *Abused Chil-*

dren in America: Victims of Official Neglect. Washington, DC: U.S. Government Printing Office, 1987.

______ . *No Place to Call Home: Discarded Children in America.* Washington, DC: U.S. Government Printing Office, 1989.

______ . *Youth and the Justice System: Can We Intervene Earlier?* Washington, DC: U.S. Government Printing Office, 1984.

Shelton, P. "Separation and Treatment of Child-Abusing Families." *Family Therapy* 9, no. 1 (1982): 53-59.

Smith, C.P., D.J. Berkman, and W.M. Fraser. *A Preliminary National Assessment of Child Abuse and Neglect and the Juvenile Justice System: The Shadows of Distress.* Washington, DC: U.S. Department of Justice, Office of Juvenile Justice and Delinquency Prevention, 1980.

Smith, C.P., T.E. Black, and F.R. Campbell. *A National Assessment of Case Disposition and Classification in the Juvenile Justice System: Inconsistent Labeling.* Vol. 1, *Process Description and Summary.* Washington, DC: Office of Juvenile Justice and Delinquency Prevention, 1980.

Smith, S.R. "The Changing Politics of Child Welfare Services: New Roles for the Government and the Nonprofit Sectors." *Child Welfare* 68, no. 3 (1989): 289-299.

Steinberg, L.D., R. Catalano, and D. Dooley. "Economic Antecedents of Child Abuse and Neglect." *Child Development* 52 (1981): 975-985.

Straker, G., and R.S. Jacobson. "Aggression, Emotional Maladjustment, and Empathy in the Abused Child." *Developmental Psychology* 17 (1981): 762-765.

Straus, M.A. "The Conflict Tactics Scales: An Evaluation and New Data on Validity, Reliability, Norms, and Scoring Methods." Paper presented at the National Council on Family Relations, Durham, NH, October, 1987.

Straus, M.A. "Measuring Intrafamily Conflict and Violence: The Conflict Tactics (CT) Scales." *Journal of Marriage and the Family* 41 (1979): 75-88.

Subramanian, K. "Reducing Child Abuse Through Respite Center Intervention." *Child Welfare* 64, no. 5 (1985): 501-509.

Swire, M., and F. Kavaler. "Health Supervision of Children in Foster Care." *Child Welfare* 57, no. 6 (1978): 563-569.

Tatara, T., P.R. Casey, K.L. Nazar, F.K. Richmond, R. Diethorn, and T. Chapmond. "Evaluation of Independent-Living Programs." *Child Welfare* 67, no. 6 (1988): 609-623.

Terrell, P. "Purchasing Social Services." In *Encyclopedia of Social Work,* 18th ed., ed. National Association of Social Workers, 434-442. Silver Spring, MD: NASW, 1987.

U.S. Advisory Board on Child Abuse and Neglect. *Child Abuse and Neglect: Critical First Steps in Response to a National Emergency.* Washington, DC: U.S. Government Printing Office, 1990.

U.S. Department of Health, Education, and Welfare, Office of Education. "Education of Handicapped Children: Implementation of Part B of the Education of the Handicapped Act." *Federal Register* 42, no. 63 (August 23, 1977), 42478.

Walker, C.E., and B.L. Bonner. *The Physically and Sexually Abused Child: Evaluation and Treatment.* New York: Pergamon, 1988.

Webster-Stratton, C. "Comparison of Abusive and Nonabusive Families with Conduct-Disordered Children." *American Journal of Orthopsychiatry* 55, no. 1 (1985): 59-69.

Weissman, M.M., and E.S. Paykel. *The Depressed Woman: A Study of Social Relationships.* Chicago: University of Chicago Press, 1974.

Wells, S.E. *At-Risk Youth: Identification, Programs, and Recommendations.* Englewood, CO: Teacher Ideas Press, 1990.

Widom, C.S. "Child Abuse, Neglect, and Adult Behavior: Research Design and Findings on Criminality, Violence and Child Abuse." *American Journal of Orthopsychiatry* 59 (1989): 355-367.

Wodarski, J.S., P.D. Kurtz, J.M. Gaudin, Jr., and P.T. Howing. "Maltreatment and the School-Age Child: Major Academic, Socioemotional and Adaptive Outcomes." *Social Work* 35 (1990): 506-513.

Wolfe, D.A., J. Aragona, K. Kaufman, and J. Sandler. "The Importance of Adjudication in the Treatment of Child Abusers: Some Preliminary Findings." *Child Abuse and Neglect* 4 (1980): 127-135.

Wolfe, D.A., P. Jaffe, S.K. Wilson, and L. Zak. "Children of Battered Women: The Relation of Child Behavior to Family Violence and Maternal Stress." *Journal of Consulting and Clinical Psychology* 53 (1985): 657-665.

Wolff, S. "Social and Family Background of Preschool Children with Behaviour Disorders Attending a Child Guidance Clinic." *Journal of Child Psychology and Psychiatry* 2 (1961): 260-268.

Wolock, I. "Contracting as a People-Processing Mechanism in a Public Child-Welfare Agency." In *Services for Sale: Purchasing Health and Human Services,* 200-213. New Brunswick, NJ: Rutgers University Press, 1989.

Wolock, I., and B. Horowitz. "Child Maltreatment and Maternal Deprivation Among AFDC-Recipient Families." *Social Service Review* 53 (1979): 530-543.

Yarrow, M.R., P.M. Scott, and C. Waxler. "Learning Concern for Others." *Developmental Psychology* 8 (1973): 240-260.

Author Index

Subject Index

Numbers in italics refer to tables and figures.